The Health Care Industry

The Health Care Industry

A Primer for Board Members

DENNIS D. POINTER
STEPHEN J. WILLIAMS

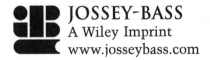

JOSSEY-BASS
A Wiley Imprint
www.josseybass.com

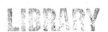
Published by Jossey-Bass
A Wiley Imprint
989 Market Street, San Francisco, CA 94103-1741   www.josseybass.com

Jossey-Bass books and products are available through most bookstores. To contact Jossey-Bass directly call our Customer Care Department within the U.S. at 800-956-7739, outside the U.S. at 317-572-3986 or fax 317-572-4002.

Jossey-Bass also publishes its books in a variety of electronic formats. Some content that appears in print may not be available in electronic books.

Library of Congress Cataloging-in-Publication Data

Pointer, Dennis Dale.
  The health care industry: a primer for board members/Dennis D. Pointer, Stephen J. Williams.—1st ed.
    p.; cm.
Includes bibliographical references and index.
  ISBN 0-7879-6721-1 (alk. paper)
  1. Medical care—United States. 2. Medical policy—United States. 3. Health services administration—United States.
  [DNLM: 1. Health Services—United States. 2. Health Services Administration—United States. 3. Insurance, Health—United States. W 84 AA1 P686h 2003] I. Williams, Stephen J. (Stephen Joseph), date. II. Title.
  RA395.A3P58 2003
  362.1'0973—dc22

                                              2003016269

Printed in the United States of America
FIRST EDITION
HB Printing   10 9 8 7 6 5 4 3 2 1

CONTENTS

LIST OF TABLES AND FIGURES

Tables

Figures

To you, board members—the leaders and
the mainstay of our health care system.
Your dedication and work make a difference!

PREFACE

How well you fulfill your responsibilities as a board member ultimately depends on how much you know. Governance is not a "competence-free zone."

Your board's decisions and actions have a huge impact on the organization, its medical staff and employees, and most important on your community. Significant and complex issues flow through the boardroom at a blistering pace. To deal with them effectively, and to decide and act with wisdom, you must understand context—how health care services are organized, financed, and provided. *The Health Care Industry: A Primer for Board Members* helps you acquire this fundamental prerequisite of enlightened and empowered directorship, and do so without having to plow through a mountain of books and articles.

Although targeted at board members, both new and long-tenured, this book is of value to anyone seeking an introduction to the characteristics, structure, and functioning of the U.S. health care industry. It is organized as follows:

- Chapter One is a general overview of the health care industry: the "big picture" of one of the economy's largest, and most important, sectors; a little history to bring some perspective; the underlying causes of health and disease; characteristics of health care organization boards; and the nature of governance responsibilities and roles.
- Chapter Two deals with organizations that provide health care services: ambulatory care, the "front line" of the system; hospitals; long-term care and mental health facilities; health systems; and public health agencies.

- Chapter Three addresses finances: the industry's changing economic dynamics; where the money comes from and goes; types of health plans; voluntary (private) health insurance; governmental programs (Medicare and Medicaid); and health maintenance organizations.

- Chapter Four focuses on the people who provide care: who they are; their characteristics; and how they are trained.

- Chapter Five forwards some predictions about the health care industry's future and the challenges they pose.

- Appendix A is a health care glossary. Whenever you encounter an unfamiliar term, concept, or acronym in the book, consult this reference.

- Appendix B offers a description of medical specialties and subspecialties.

- Appendix C puts forward recommendations for learning more about the industry.

- The References section is a list of sources drawn upon in this book.

We concentrate on the basics. Complex issues are simplified and much is left unsaid. But after reading this book you will have a solid grounding for understanding the industry in which your organization and board function.

Dennis D. Pointer, Ph.D.
President
Dennis D. Pointer & Associates
Seattle, Washington
(206) 632-6066
dennis.pointer@comcast.net

Austin Ross Professor of Health Care
*   Management*
Department of Health Services
School of Public Health and
*   Community Medicine*
University of Washington
Seattle, Washington
dpointer@u.washington.edu

Vice President and Partner
American Governance and
*   Leadership Group, LLC*
dpointer@Americangovernance.com

Stephen J. Williams, Sc.D.
Professor and Head
Division of Health Services
Graduate School of Public Health
San Diego State University
San Diego, California
(619) 594-4433
swilliam@mail.sdsu.edu

ABOUT THE AUTHORS

Dennis D. Pointer is one of the nation's foremost governance consultants, speakers, and writers. He is the author of more than seventy articles and seven books, among them *Really Governing* and *Board Work* (both winners of the James A. Hamilton Book of the Year Award from the American College of Healthcare Executives); *Getting to Great: Principles of Health Care Organization Governance;* and *The High Performance Board.* He has been the chair or a member of more than twenty boards.

His firm, Dennis D. Pointer & Associates, provides governance consulting, retreat facilitation, assessment, and design and development services. DDP&A has worked with more than 450 clients, including health systems and hospitals, nonprofit organizations, commercial corporations, and government agencies. He is also vice president and partner, American Governance and Leadership Group, which provides board education and development services to health care organizations.

Pointer is Austin Ross Professor, Department of Health Services, University of Washington School of Public Health and Community Medicine. He has held two previous endowed chairs: the John J. Hanlon Professorship of Health Services Research and Policy, at the Graduate School of Public Health, San Diego State University (1991–2002 and currently emeritus); and the Arthur Graham Glasgow Chair of Health Services Management at the Medical College of Virginia (1986–1991). From 1975 to 1986, he was affiliated with the University of California, Los Angeles, where he served as professor and chair of the Department of Health Services Management, School of Public Health; and as associate director of the UCLA Medical

Center. During his tenure at UCLA, he was a Senior Fellow at the RAND Corporation. Pointer has held faculty appointments at the University of Iowa, the Mount Sinai School of Medicine, and the Baruch School of Management of the City University of New York, in addition to having served as associate director of the Department of Teaching Hospitals, Association of American Medical Colleges. He received his Ph.D. from the University of Iowa.

Pointer is a recipient of the Foster G. McGaw Medal of Excellence in Health Administration, Education, and Research; he has been a Dozor Distinguished Visiting Professor of Medical Administration at Ben Gurion University (Beer Sheva, Israel).

Stephen J. Williams is a nationally recognized educator and author in the area of health services. He has written more than seventy-five articles and twenty-five books, among which is the leading textbook on the nation's health care system, *Introduction to Health Services* (with Paul Torrens). He has also coauthored the most popular textbook on group practice management.

Williams has been the principal investigator on more than $2 million of federal and private research grants and has served as a consultant to numerous health care organizations, associations, and governmental agencies.

Williams is professor of public health and head of the Division of Health Services Administration in the Graduate School of Public Health, San Diego State University. He was previously associate director of the University of Washington's program in health services administration. He is editor of the Delmar Series in Health Services and was a series editor for John Wiley and Sons. He received his graduate training at the Massachusetts Institute of Technology's Sloan School of Management and the Harvard University School of Public Health.

The Health Care Industry

CHAPTER 1

Foundations

Health care is one of our economy's largest industries; it contributes significantly to the nation's competitiveness and productivity in addition to enhancing citizens' well-being and quality of life.

AT A GLANCE

The industry is a complex mix of government; nonprofit and commercial organizations; and individual efforts to finance, provide, and regulate health care services. Major industry sectors include:

- *Financing sector* Organizations that reimburse health care providers, such as the Centers for Medicare and Medicaid Services (a federal agency), state workers' compensation programs, health insurance companies, and health maintenance organizations
- *Institutional providers* Organizations that provide personal health care services, such as physician offices, medical groups, hospitals, mental health facilities, nursing homes, and home health agencies
- *Individual providers* Professionals who offer personal health care services, such as physicians, dentists, chiropractors, nurses, pharmacists, and psychologists
- *Public health agencies* Government agencies that promote health and prevent disease in populations, such as the Centers for Disease Control and Prevention and state/local health departments

- *Enablers* Organizations that support and facilitate the provision of health services, such as trade and professional associations (for example, the American Hospital Association and American Medical Association), special interest groups (American Heart Association), research organizations (National Institutes of Health), and educational institutions (medical and nursing schools)
- *Suppliers* Organizations that provide products and services, such as pharmaceutical manufacturers, hospital supply and equipment companies, and consulting firms
- *Regulators* Government agencies and private organizations that regulate health care institutions and professionals, such as medical specialty societies, state licensing boards, state insurance departments, and the Joint Commission on Accreditation of Healthcare Organizations

This classification is not precise; definitions of who belongs where are often fuzzy and membership in the various sectors can overlap.

Table 1.1 is an overview of the U.S. health care industry's magnitude and scope.

SOME HISTORY

The country's first hospital opened its doors in 1756. Over the past 250 years, hospitals have undergone many profound changes; the key stages are summarized in Table 1.2. Each stage entailed its own challenges, and the group best equipped to deal with them exercised the greatest power.

Refuge Stage

This stage spans approximately 170 years, from the mid-1700s to the late 1920s.

Pennsylvania Hospital, the nation's first, opened in 1756; New York Hospital, the second, was founded in 1776. It was not until the mid-1850s that there were more than a handful of organizations devoted to providing inpatient health care. A survey conducted in 1873 identified only 178 hospitals. Medical knowledge was primitive and physicians could do little of

The Health Care Industry: A Primer

Table 1.1. Overview of the U.S. Health Care Industry, 2002

National Health Care Expenditures

Per year	$1.3 trillion
Per day	$3.6 billion
Per hour	$148 million
Per minute	$2.5 million
Per second	$36,500
Per person	$4,000
Percentage of gross domestic product	13
Percentage from government funds	43
Percentage from private funds	57
Percentage spent on the provision of personal health care services	87
Spent on prescription drugs	$122 billion

Source of Funds	**Percentage**
Total expenditures from:	
Out-of-pocket (individuals)	17
Private health insurance	34
Other private sources	5
Federal government	33
State governments	11

Health Insurance

With no coverage:	
Number of individuals	41 million
Percentage of the population under age 65	17
Percentage of population that has coverage through:	
Private health insurance (those under age 65)	72
Private health insurance provided by employer (those under age 65)	67
Enrollment in a health maintenance organization (those under age 65)	34
Medicare	14
Medicaid	9

General, Short-Stay Hospitals

Organizations	5,800
Beds	1 million

(*Continued*)

Table 1.1. Overview of the
U.S. Health Care Industry, 2002, Cont'd

Average beds occupied	66%
Average hospital size	170 beds
Annual inpatient admissions	35 million
Average inpatient stay	6.8 days
Annual (hospital) outpatient visits	85 million
Annual (hospital) emergency room visits	108 million
Annual expenditures	$412 billion

Nursing Homes

Organizations	17,000
Beds	1.8 million
Average beds occupied	82%
Average daily residents	1.5 million
Annual expenditures	$92 billion

Mental and Behavioral Health

Psychiatric hospitals	580
Psychiatric units in general hospitals	1,700
Annual expenditures	$33 billion

Personnel

Total health care industry workforce	12 million
Percentage of all working adults	9%

Physicians

Number (active)	690,000
Annual office visits	824 million
Annual expenditures	$286 billion

Other Health Care Personnel

Registered nurses	2.3 million
Pharmacists	208,000
Dentists	168,000
Physical therapists	144,000
Speech therapists	97,000
Podiatrists	11,000

Table 1.2. Evolution of the U.S. Health Care Industry

Stage	Challenge	Greatest Power or Influence
Refuge	Create institutions and raise funds; *provide care*	Board
Physician workshop	Achieve efficacy; expand capacities and competencies; *produce cures*	Physicians
Business	Improve organizational effectiveness and efficiency; *rationalize*	Management
System	Improve organizational competitiveness; *combine and integrate*	Shared and collaborative

value; treatments were primarily supportive and many were detrimental. Those patients able to pay received care in their homes, because hospitals were very dangerous places because of infections.

This was a period of institution building. Hospitals were new types of organizations with missions different from that of almshouses (warehouses for the poor, aged, and infirm), from which they evolved. Their survival depended on gaining community acceptance and raising funds. Nearly all hospitals were charitable organizations, and the money needed to create and operate them was donated.

Hospital boards, composed of a community's social and financial elite, were the only groups capable of performing these critical tasks. Consequently, they possessed power and exercised influence hard to imagine today.

By 1909, there were forty-three hundred hospitals; in 1923, there were more than seven thousand. This growth, plus dramatic advances in biomedical science, precipitated the next stage and significantly altered the locus of power in hospitals.

Physician Workshop Stage

This stage began in the early 1930s and concluded in the 1960s. With the task of institution building complete, hospitals sought to improve their clinical efficacy. Physicians acquired power by controlling the knowledge, skills, and technologies that transformed hospitals from offering supportive care to producing cures.

Basic biomedical knowledge, accumulating throughout the middle and late 1800s, reached critical mass in the first decades of the twentieth century. Hospitals were revolutionized in three ways. First, because infections could be partially controlled, hospitals became much safer places. Second, treatments were developed that could alter the course of disease. Third, thanks to the development of anesthesia, surgery could be safely and effectively performed. The late John Knowles, M.D., former CEO of Massachusetts General Hospital, observed, "It was not until about 1915 that the average patient with a common disease entering the average hospital, being treated by the typical physician had a better than 50/50 chance of benefiting from the experience."

Those able to pay began seeking care in hospitals. Physicians controlled the knowledge base and flow of patients on which hospitals relied. Accordingly, hospital success became far more dependent on physicians than on trustees. Boards and administrators established the setting and resources employed by physicians; hospitals became doctors' workshops.

Because all but the simplest cases were treated by them, hospitals became the epicenter of America's health care system.

Business Stage

This stage ran from the mid-1960s through the 1980s. To provide physicians what they required to practice, hospitals had to become more business-oriented. As a consequence, far better managerial talent and systems were needed.

Exponentially expanding medical knowledge and skills increased the hospital's size, scope, and complexity. As medical practice became more specialized, the amount and sophistication of facilities, equipment, and support personnel increased dramatically. Additionally, the growth of private health insurance, combined with enactment of Medicare and Medicaid in the mid-1960s, infused huge amounts of money into the industry and increased the regulations with which hospitals had to comply.

The most important challenges facing hospitals were managing growth and improving operational effectiveness and efficiency. Professional health care managers acquired power and influence in the process; they moved from being servants of the board (in the refuge stage) and lieutenants of the medical staff (in the physician workshop stage) to full-fledged executives responsible for directing the affairs of complex, multimillion dollar organizations.

At the beginning of this stage, a little more than 5 percent of the nation's gross domestic product was spent on health care; by 1985 the figure was 10 percent. Health care was now big business.

System Stage

This stage began in the mid-1980s and continues to the present day. Three developments define it: increasing consolidation, greater competition, and dramatic changes in the nature and form of payment.

First, health care organizations consolidated. For example, many hospitals merged and then combined with physician practices, nursing homes, and health insurance plans. Health systems were created.

Second, the industry became far more competitive. Not only did health systems and hospitals compete with each other but they also began competing with their own medical staffs, insurance companies, and managed care organizations.

Third, change occurred in how providers were paid, as purchasers sought to control double-digit inflation in their health care expenditures. Throughout the 1960s and 1970s, hospitals were reimbursed on the basis of their charges or incurred costs; physicians received fees or customary charges. In the 1980s, hospitals started being paid rates that were set prospectively (irrespective of their incurred costs), assuming some of the financial risk associated with providing services. Additionally, doctors, hospitals, and other health care organizations had to cooperate in order to offer the full spectrum of services demanded by purchasers.

The key challenge faced by health systems was to form and manage a diverse array of enterprises and relationships that would allow them to compete in markets undergoing significant change. This required high levels of coordination among boards, between management teams and physicians, and across organizations. As a consequence, power and influence was increasingly shared.

HEALTH AND DISEASE

Health is defined by the World Health Organization (WHO) as complete physical, mental, and social well-being, not merely the absence of disease or infirmity.

Disease impairs the functioning of a person. It can be caused by genetic flaws; the natural, preprogrammed and progressive breakdown in biological systems that increases with age; external agents (chemical, biologic, radiological); and trauma (such as accidents).

A person's health is affected by genetic predisposition, age, context (including such things as income level, education, housing, nutrition, sanitation, environment), and the use of health care services. These factors are listed here in decreasing order of importance; genetics, age, and context have a far greater impact on a person's health status than the amount and type of health care services consumed. The reason is that health care services primarily come into play only after the horse is out of the barn, when an illness or condition has already occurred. Meanwhile, other factors affect the probability that an illness or condition will appear in the first place.

Table 1.3 portrays selected indicators of Americans' health and disease status.

HEALTH SERVICE NEED, DEMAND, AND UTILIZATION

What affects the utilization of health care services? Figure 1.1 depicts the key relationships.

Table 1.3. U.S. Health and Disease Status

Infant Mortality Rate (Deaths per 1,000 Live Births)

White	6
Black	14
Hispanic	6
American Indian	9
Infant mortality ranking of the United States compared to selected other countries	27th

Life Expectancy at Birth

Males	74 years
Females	79 years
Life expectancy ranking of the United States compared to selected other countries	20th

Age-Adjusted Death Rate (Deaths per 100,000 Persons, Adjusted for Differences in Age)

White	860
Black	1148
American Indian	716
Hispanic	601

Population with Limitation of Activity Caused by Chronic Conditions

	Percentage
Under 18	6
18 to 44	6
45 to 54	12
55 to 64	20
65 to 74	26
Over 74	45

(*Continued*)

Table 1.3. U.S. Health and Disease Status, Cont'd

Index of Respondent-Reported Overall Health Status
(Lower Scores Are Healthier)

Total	9
Poor	21
Near poor	15
Nonpoor	6
Persons (age 20–74) with hypertension	24%
Persons (age 20–74) with an unhealthy weight	58%
Children (age 6–19) who are overweight	11%
Number of deaths annually	2,391,000

Cause of Death	Percentage of Total
Heart disease	31
Cancer	23
Stroke	7
Chronic obstructive pulmonary disease	5
Accidents	4
Pneumonia and influenza	4
Diabetes	3
Suicide	1
Kidney disease	1
Chronic liver disease	1

The factors and stages are:

- *Need:* recognition of an underlying abnormal condition judged to warrant care and treatment
- *Demand:* motivation and the means to seek care
- *Utilization:* consumption of health care services

> **Figure 1.1. Key Determinants of Health Care Service Utilization**
>
> Physical, biological, or mental abnormality
> (perceived or actual)
>
> ↓
>
> Need for health care services
>
> ↓
>
> Demand for health care services
>
> ↓
>
> Utilization of health care services

The presence of a disease or condition does not necessarily cause need. Need may not precipitate demand, and demand may not result in utilization.

Condition → demand   *Example:* A person may have a condition that goes undetected because it is asymptomatic. Or the underlying condition may not be defined as a disease (as was the case for many mental disorders in the early part of the last century).

Need → demand   *Example:* Individuals can demand care without needing it (as in the case of hypochondriacs). They also might need care and not demand it because the condition is thought to be inconsequential.

Demand → utilization   The conversion of demand into consumption of health care services is most affected by the two-sided coin of access: individual wherewithal (knowledge, time, and money); and by how health services are organized, financed, and provided (industry structure and functioning).

A host of factors have been shown to affect the demand for, and utilization of, health care services. Here are a few important ones:

- Age
- Insurance coverage
- Race/ethnicity
- Number and distribution of providers
- Education level
- Provider referral patterns
- Income level
- Attitudes and beliefs

As an illustration, Table 1.4 presents data on ambulatory care usage (total doctor's office, hospital emergency room, and home health visits per year) and how it varies by population group.

BOARDS AND GOVERNANCE

There are approximately six thousand hospital and health system boards, with about one hundred thousand people serving on them. Here is some basic information.

Board Composition

Health Systems

The typical health care system board is composed of fourteen members: one inside director (who holds a board seat *ex officio* by virtue of a full-time administrative position), two medical staff directors (physicians who hold board seats because of their

Hospitals

The average hospital board is composed of fifteen members: one insider, three medical staff directors, and eleven outsiders.

Table 1.4. Percentage of Individuals with No Doctor's Office, Hospital Emergency Room, or Home Health Visits During the Past Twelve Months

Category	Percentage
All persons	17
Age:	
Under 18	12
18 to 44	23
45 to 64	15
65 and over	8
Gender:	
Male	22
Female	12
Race:	
White	16
Black	17
American Indian	21
Asian	20
Hispanic	unavailable
Economic status:	
Poor	22
Near poor	21
Nonpoor	14
Under age 65, health insurance coverage:	
Insured (private)	14
Insured (Medicaid)	14
Uninsured	37
Geographic region:	
Northeast	12
Midwest	15
South	18
West	20
Residence:	
Urban	17
Rural	17

membership on the medical staff), and eleven outside directors (board members who are neither inside nor medical staff directors).

Eighty-two percent of systems limit the number of consecutive terms a director can serve (the median is three terms).

Fifty percent of hospitals have term limits (the median is three terms).

Twenty-one percent of system directors are female; 94 percent of system boards have at least one female member.

Eighteen percent of hospital directors are female; only 6 percent of hospitals have no female members.

Minorities hold 7 percent of system board seats; 5 percent are Black, 1 percent are Hispanic, 0.7 percent are Asian, and 0.1 percent are Native American. Thirty-seven percent of system boards have at least one minority member.

Minorities compose 7 percent of hospital directors; 6 percent are Black, 0.7 percent are Hispanic, and 0.3 percent are Asian. Fifty percent of hospital boards have no racial or ethnic minority members.

Board Functioning

Health Systems

Ninety-six percent of systems have a person assigned to provide staff support to the board; 10 percent of systems have a designated board coordinator. Staff support to the board is from an executive assistant in 60 percent of systems; this person is typically attached to the office of the president or CEO. On

Hospitals

Ninety-four percent of hospitals have a person assigned to extend staff support to the board. In hospitals with governance staff support, 15 percent have a formally designated board coordinator; 80 percent use an executive or administrative assistant or secretary, and 5 percent assign a average, about one-quarter FTE (full-time-equivalent) is devoted to board staffing.

System directors spend on average twenty-three hours per year involved in formal educational activities related to their roles.

Eighteen percent of systems compensate their directors.

Thirty-eight percent of system boards meet monthly, 40 percent meet every other month, and 18 percent meet quarterly.

The typical system board meeting lasts three and one-half hours; on average, 11 percent of members are absent.

member of the management team. On average, one-half FTE is allocated to board staffing.

The typical hospital director spends about seventeen hours per year involved in governance education.

Ten percent of hospitals compensate their directors. In the vast majority of instances, the amount of compensation is nominal (less than $1,000 per year).

Fifty-six percent of hospital boards meet monthly, 19 percent meet every other month, and 8 percent meet quarterly.

The average hospital board meeting lasts two hours; 13 percent of members are typically absent.

The most common system and hospital standing committees are executive, finance, planning or strategy, quality or credentialing, nominating, and audit.

Eighty-six percent of health system board chairpersons are outsiders, 6 percent are medical staff directors, and 8 percent are insiders.

Seventy-four percent of system board chairpersons are male and 2 percent are minorities.

For hospital board chairpersons, the corresponding figures are 94 percent, 4 percent, and 2 percent.

Among hospital board chairpersons 79 percent are male and 2 percent are minorities.

Governance Work

The fundamental obligation of all boards is to represent an organization's owners, ensuring that resources and capacities are deployed in ways that benefit them. In for-profit health care organizations, the owners are stockholders; in nonprofits, they are stakeholders (such as the community); and in governmental facilities they are constituents (voters).

To meet this obligation, a board must discharge four core responsibilities.

1. Determining *ends*: formulating the organization's vision and mission, specifying its key goals, and ensuring that strategies (developed by management) will lead to accomplishing goals and fulfilling the vision and mission

2. Ensuring a high level of *management* performance: recruiting and selecting the CEO; specifying CEO performance expectations; assessing the CEO's performance and contributions; adjusting the CEO's compensation; and, if the need arises, terminating the CEO's employment

3. Ensuring the *quality* of patient care: appointing or reappointing members of the medical staff and determining their privileges; making sure that necessary quality, utilization, and risk measurement and management systems are in place and functioning effectively; and assessing the quality of care provided

4. Ensuring *financial* health: specifying financial objectives; determining if management-devised budgets are aligned with financial objectives and to the organization's key goals, vision, and mission; monitoring and evaluating financial performance and outcomes; and making sure that financial controls are in place and the organization's financial statements accurately reflect its financial status

To fulfill these responsibilities, a board must have the right structure, composition, and infrastructure.

Structure is how governance work is subdivided and coordinated within the organization; it deals with such things as board size, the number and type of committees, and (in systems) the number of boards and their relationships. *Composition* focuses on board members—their characteristics, knowledge, skills, perspectives, and experience. *Infrastructure* includes the resources and systems that support the performance of governance work.

CHAPTER 2

Health Care Organizations and Services

This chapter examines health care organizations (HCOs) and the services they provide, of which there are two types: personal and public. *Personal HCOs* provide services that are consumed by, and affect, individuals, such as a physician office visit or an inpatient hospital stay. *Public HCOs* provide services that are targeted at and affect populations, such as sanitation, drinking water fluoridation, and the control of communicable diseases.

According to the U.S. Census Bureau, there are approximately 470,000 establishments that provide personal health care services. Two-thirds are physician and dentists' offices; only 2 percent are hospitals, although they account for about 40 percent of the industry's employment. The distribution of health care establishments is noted in Table 2.1.

DISTINCTIVE CHARACTERISTICS

Organizations providing personal health care services have some distinctive characteristics:

• *Service offering.* HCOs provide services, not products. Services are intangibles that are purchased, produced, and used simultaneously. Karl Marx

**Table 2.1. Distribution of Establishments
Providing Personal Health Care Services**

Type	Percentage of All Establishments
Physician offices	41
Dentist offices	25
Offices of other health care practitioners	19
Nursing homes	6
Medical and dental laboratories	4
Other	3
Hospitals	2

(in *Das Capital*), displaying unusual humor, described them as something you can buy but can't drop on your foot. Health care services cannot be stored; capacity that goes unused (such as an unoccupied hospital bed) is lost forever. As a consequence, demand must be either accurately predicted or carefully controlled for an HCO's resources to be productively deployed. Additionally, services (particularly health care) are custom-designed while they are being produced; their form and content varies from client to client.

• *Importance.* Health care services fulfill basic needs rather than peripheral wants and desires, and so they are critical. They have a huge impact on clients' quality of life (and often their survival); when needed, few offerings are as important.

• *Intimacy.* Health care services focus on the self. They are physically and psychologically invasive, and they are provided when a person is most threatened, frightened, and vulnerable. As a consequence, their use has a high emotional and spiritual charge.

• *Consumption is a right.* Because of their criticality, access to basic health care services is typically guaranteed irrespective of a person's circumstances or ability to pay. Government has the responsibility of ensuring life, liberty, and the pursuit of happiness; health care services enable two of these three rights.

- *Purchasers and customers.* For most goods, those who purchase also consume. This is often not the case for health care services. They are used by individuals but typically purchased (paid for), in whole or in part, by employers and government. Because of this, providers must respond to two sets of potentially conflicting expectations and demands, one from purchasers and another from customers.

- *Insurance.* The use of most health care services is insured. Patients make few if any out-of-pocket expenditures at the point where they consume care. Consequently, there are few immediate economic incentives to limit use.

- *Complexity.* The process of producing health care services is complex because the workings of the human body are incompletely understood and the store of knowledge regarding diagnostic and therapeutic technology is vast.

- *Professional workers.* The health care workforce is highly professionalized; professionals are characterized by extensive, intensive, and lengthy training. Far more so than in other occupations, professionals are granted (through such mechanisms as licensing laws) and expect or demand a high degree of autonomy, discretion, and control over their work and the context in which they practice.

- *Ownership and control of key factor inputs.* Organizations typically employ the most critical personnel needed to produce their products and services (examples are airlines hiring pilots, flight attendants, and mechanics; and restaurants employing chefs). HCOs are a notable exception. Most do not employ physicians, even though the medical staff has tremendous influence over an HCO's operation (who will be admitted; the course of treatment; the amount and type of resources employed; and as a consequence costs, productivity, and margins).

- *Error tolerances.* Mistakes made in HCOs often have negative and irreversible consequences, jeopardizing well-being and causing death.

- *Operational time frame.* Most HCOs operate twenty-four hours a day, seven days per week, 365 days a year; they never close, must be continuously staffed, and have no down time.

AMBULATORY CARE

Ambulatory care is the term used to describe services provided to noninstitutionalized patients whose treatment does not require an overnight stay in a health care facility.

Ranging from quite complex to routine, ambulatory care is the backbone of the nation's personal health care system, for several reasons. First, an ambulatory care visit is the initial point of contact between patients and other system components. Second, the vast majority of health care is provided on an ambulatory basis. Third, an increasing number of diagnostic and therapeutic procedures, once done only during an inpatient hospital stay, are now being carried out in ambulatory care settings owing to dramatic advances in technology, changes in financial incentives, and demands for greater patient convenience.

Access to, and use of, ambulatory care varies considerably with an individual's social, economic, and demographic characteristics (see Table 2.2). Ambulatory care is offered in a variety of settings by many types of health care professionals.

Illustrative Sites	Illustrative Professionals
Professional offices	Physicians
Clinics	Physician assistants
Group practices	Nurses
Hospital outpatient departments	Dentists
Emergency rooms	Pharmacists
Urgent care facilities	Chiropractors
Same-day surgery centers	Podiatrists

Table 2.2. Adults (18–64 Years of Age) with No Regular Source of Care

Category	Percentage
All	18
Age	
18 to 24	27
25 to 44	20
45 to 54	12
55 to 64	9
Gender	
Male	24
Female	12
Race	
White	17
Black	19
Hispanic	31
Insurance status	
Insured	11
Uninsured	47

Community health centers

Student health clinics

Occupational health programs (located on employers' sites)

Home health and visiting nurse agencies

Physical therapists

Optometrists

Occupational therapists

Psychologists

Clinical social workers

The best information on ambulatory care is collected through the National Ambulatory Care Survey conducted by the National Center for Health

Statistics. The most recent survey (2000) focuses only on physician services. Here are some facts:

- During the year, there were 824 million physician visits, an average of three per person.
- The percentage distribution of all visits by physician specialty was general and family practice 24 percent; internal medicine 15 percent; pediatrics 13 percent; obstetrics and gynecology 8 percent; orthopedic surgery 6 percent; ophthalmology 5 percent; and all others 29 percent.
- People who had seen the physician previously accounted for 86 percent of all visits.
- Physicians were seen in 96 percent of all visits.
- Sixty percent of patient-physician contacts were one to fifteen minutes in length.
- About half of all visits were scheduled because of specific symptoms.
- The most frequently cited reasons for visits (in order of magnitude) were follow-up care, cough or throat condition, routine prenatal care, postoperative care, well-baby examination, vision dysfunction, ear ache or infection, back problem, joint problem, and fever and skin rash.
- Thirty-five percent of all visits were for acute problems; this increased to 50 percent in patients under fifteen years of age.
- At least one therapeutic or preventive service was ordered or provided during 35 percent of all visits.
- Sixty-six percent of visits resulted in prescription of pharmaceuticals.
- The source of payment for visits was private insurance (57 percent); Medicare (20 percent); Medicaid (9 percent); self-pay (9 percent)); workers' compensation (2 percent); no charge (1 percent), or other (about 7 percent).

- Thirty percent of visits were by patients with some form of HMO coverage.
- One-third of physicians do not accept charity patients, 10 percent do not accept new Medicare patients, and 22 percent do not accept new Medicaid patients.
- More than two-thirds of all visits were to physicians engaged in some form of group practice.

Throughout most of the twentieth century, solo practice physicians provided most office-based ambulatory services. Solo practice consists of an individual physician, generally assisted by several clinical and administrative personnel. Group practice involves the collective effort of three or more physicians, often complemented by other health care professionals, who share resources (facilities, personnel, systems), pool expenses and income, and collaborate in the care of patients.

Since the 1970s, there has been a pronounced shift from solo to group practice. This is due to the increasing complexity of medicine; the administrative burdens imposed by patient billing, filing insurance claims, and negotiating managed care contracts, and the increasing cost of setting up and running a practice. Between 1969 and 1999, the number of physician groups grew from about six thousand to twenty-one thousand (a threefold increase); during the same period the number of physicians in groups increased from forty thousand to 214,000 (a fivefold increase).

There are two principle types of group practices. In single-specialty groups, physicians are members of the same medical or surgical specialty. Multispecialty group practices are composed of physicians representing various specialties. About 70 percent of physician groups are single-specialty and the remainder multispecialty.

As is portrayed in Figure 2.1, groups vary considerably by size. Although 95 percent of physician groups have fewer than twenty-five members, 45 percent of the total number of physicians practicing in groups belong to those that exceed twenty-five members.

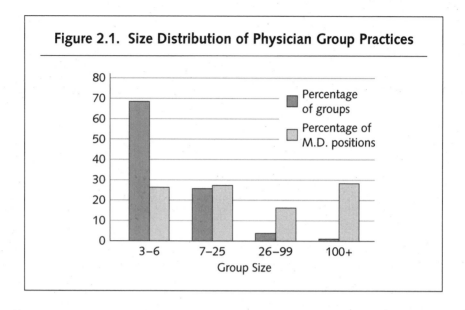

Figure 2.1. Size Distribution of Physician Group Practices

HOSPITAL CARE

Hospitals serve patients requiring at least an overnight stay. They provide intensive, round-the-clock nursing care; all other patients can be treated elsewhere.

As discussed in Chapter One, the American hospital has evolved from a repository for the poor with hopeless medical conditions to the site of our nation's most sophisticated diagnostic and therapeutic capabilities. With the increasing shift of care to ambulatory settings and other types of health care organizations (such as home health agencies and long-term care facilities), hospitals now provide the most intense services to the sickest patients requiring the greatest amount of care.

Hospitals are the heavyweights of the health care industry. Expenditures for hospital care have increased from $9 billion in 1960 to more than $400 billion in 2000 (see Figure 2.2) and now account for about one-third of all health care expenditures.

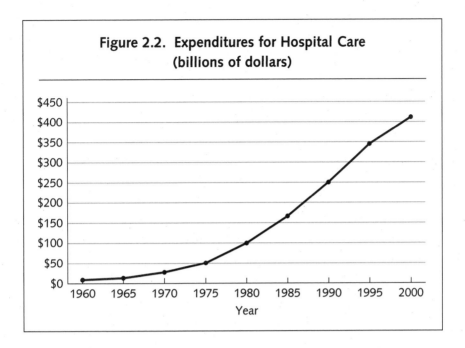

**Figure 2.2. Expenditures for Hospital Care
(billions of dollars)**

There are just under six thousand hospitals in the country with about one million hospital beds; they admit more than thirty-four million patients each year. Hospitals employ six million people.

Hospitals are typically classified by their length of stay, type of patient service, and ownership.

• *Length of stay.* Hospitals can be either short-term or long-term. Short-term hospitals treat individuals with acute problems requiring inpatient stays that average about five days; the typical community hospital is a short-stay facility. Long-term hospitals deal with chronic conditions requiring stays that can range from a month to several years; examples are psychiatric, chronic disease, and rehabilitation facilities.

• *Type of service.* General hospitals offer an array of medical and surgical services. Specialty hospitals treat a narrow range of patients—children, women, or those with a specific condition such as cancer or orthopedic problems. About 70 percent of the nation's hospitals are in the general category; the remainder are specialty hospitals.

• *Ownership.* The major classifications are nonprofit, proprietary, federal government, and state or local government.

Nonprofit (typically referred to as voluntary) hospitals are organized as 501(c)(3) tax-exempt corporations. They are "owned" by the community in which they operate, or by other charitable organizations such as religious congregations, fraternal organizations, and associations.

Proprietary (for-profit or investor-owned) hospitals are operated for the purpose of producing a return for their investors. Throughout most of the twentieth century, the typical proprietary hospital was locally owned by an individual or a group of physicians. Beginning in the 1960s, many of these institutions were bought by commercial stock corporations, which, during the eighties and nineties, increased the number of beds through building programs and by acquiring nonprofit facilities.

The distribution of hospitals and beds by ownership is displayed in Table 2.3.

When most people say "hospital," they are thinking of a nonfederal, short-term, acute care, general facility, known as a community hospital. An

Table 2.3. Distribution of U.S. Hospitals and Beds, by Ownership

Ownership	Hospitals (Number)	Hospitals (Percentage)	Beds (Number)	Beds (Percentage)
Federal	245	5	53,000	6
Nonprofit	3,003	57	583,000	66
Proprietary	749	15	110,000	13
State or local government	1,163	23	131,000	15

organization of this kind is the mainstay of the nation's health system and one of a community's most important resources. A profile of community hospitals is provided in Table 2.4.

The typical hospital is composed of four distinct, but highly interdependent, components (see Figure 2.3):

1. The *board* is responsible for governing the hospital on behalf of its "owners"—the community in a nonprofit hospital, shareholders in a proprietary hospital, or constituents in a governmental hospital.

2. *Management* is accountable to the board for running the organization on a day-to-day basis—strategically, financially, and operationally. Typically, management is thought of as carrying out board directives. However, given the complexity of the contemporary hospital, executives are board partners in formulating an organization's vision and mission, goals, objectives, and policies.

3. The *medical staff* provides, and directs provision of, clinical care within the hospital. Its members are physicians and sometimes other health care professionals (such as dentists and podiatrists), appointed by the board. In most hospitals, physicians are not employees. Rather, they are independent practitioners who use the hospital for the care of their patients.

4. The hospital's *operational component* is responsible for performing nonmedical, clinical (for example, nursing) and support ("hotel" service, administrative, technical) work. It is directly accountable to management but influenced by members of the medical staff.

Many hospitals are affiliated with, or owned by, health care systems. This type of organization is addressed in a later section of this chapter.

LONG-TERM CARE

Long-term care comprises an array of ambulatory and inpatient medical, mental-behavioral, social, and daily living support services. The primary users are individuals with temporary disabilities or chronic health problems. The first group have injuries or illnesses that impair their ability to

Table 2.4. Community Hospital Profile

Criterion	Total	Per Hospital
Hospitals	5,000	
Utilization, inpatient		
Beds	830,000	170
Admissions	32,359,000	6,500
Inpatient days	191,824,000	39,000
Average length of stay (days)	6	
Inpatient surgeries	9,540,000	1,900
Births	3,760,000	760
Utilization, outpatient		
Total outpatient visits	495,346,000	100,000
Emergency room visits	99,484,000	20,000
Outpatient surgeries	15,845,000	3,200
Personnel		
Total full-time	3,298,000	670
Total part-time	1,247,000	250
Percentage part-time	38	
Operating and financial statistics		
Gross revenue, inpatient	$436 billion	$88 million
Gross revenue, outpatient	$224 billion	$45 million
Total expenses	$335 billion	$68 million
Net margin	$16 billion	$3 million
Admissions per bed	39	
Percentage of admissions with surgeries performed	29	
Full-time employees per bed	4.0	
Part-time employees per bed	1.5	
Gross inpatient revenue per patient day	$2,300	
Inpatient revenue per admission	$13,500	
Total net revenue per admission	$11,000	
Total expense per admission	$10,000	

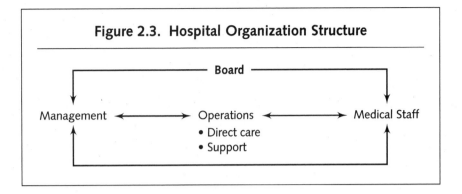

Figure 2.3. Hospital Organization Structure

function independently for a period of time but who will eventually recover; examples are those suffering from stroke, trauma, and severe bone fractures. The second group have progressively degenerative and nonreversible physical or mental conditions; examples are spinal cord injury, Alzheimer's disease, and infirmity due to aging.

Most long-term care services are consumed by older individuals. This segment of the population will continue to grow dramatically as baby boomers age. In 1990, 13 percent of the population was over the age of sixty-five; by 2030 this group will make up about 20 percent of the population. Functional disability increases with age. Additionally, approximately 125 million Americans of all ages suffer from some type of chronic illness.

Most long-term care is rendered by family members and friends in the home, supplemented with ambulatory and inpatient services:

• Monitoring and care management provided in a doctor's office or clinic
• Home visitors
• Homemaker and personal care
• Meals on Wheels
• Visiting nursing

- Adult day care
- Respite care
- Congregate care
- Independent senior housing
- Group homes
- Assisted living centers
- Nursing home care
- Ambulatory and inpatient mental/behavioral care
- Inpatient rehabilitation care
- Hospice care

As a proportion of the $1.3 trillion spent on health in 2001, the largest expenditures for long-term care are nursing homes ($117 billion, or 9 percent of the total) and home health care ($39 billion, or 3 percent).

Nursing Home Care

Nursing homes provide a mix of intermediate-level nursing and personal services on a twenty-four-hour basis to individuals who are either temporarily or permanently unable to care for themselves. The home can be either freestanding or a component of another organization (such as a hospital or retirement center) and is licensed and regulated by a state.

There are approximately seventeen thousand nursing homes, with 1.8 million beds. Here is a profile of these organizations:

- Spending on nursing home care is $92 billion, up from $40 billion in 1988.
- Expenditures for nursing home care account for 24 percent of total Medicaid spending and 5 percent of Medicare spending.
- Sixty-five percent of nursing homes are proprietary, 28 percent are nonprofit, and 7 percent are governmental.

- Fifty-six percent of nursing homes are affiliated with a chain; 24 percent are independent.
- The number of beds per facility averages 107, and the occupancy rate is about 80 percent.
- Overall, the source of a typical nursing home's revenue is 47 percent Medicaid; 12 percent Medicare; and 41 percent from private health insurance, out-of-pocket expenditures, and other.
- During the year there are 2.4 million nursing home admissions; on a typical day, there are 1.6 million nursing home residents.
- The age distribution of nursing home residents is 9 percent under sixty-five, 48 percent age sixty-five to eighty-four, and 46 percent over eighty-five.
- Residents are 25 percent male and 75 percent female; 88 percent are white, 10 percent are black, and two percent are Hispanic.
- Fifty-six percent of nursing home residents are bedfast or chair-bound; 45 percent experience dementia or have some other mental deficiency, and 51 percent are taking psychoactive medications.
- The length of stay of residents varies: less than three months, 16 percent; three to six months, 10 percent; six to twelve months, 15 percent; one to three years, 31 percent; three to five years, 14 percent; and greater than five years, 15 percent.
- The average charge for nursing home care is $3,900 per month.

Home Health Care

Home health is supportive and curative care provided to patients in their residences. Services can range from simple (housekeeping and meals) to complex (skilled nursing; physical, respiratory, and intravenous therapies).

The most important distinction among home health organizations (typically called agencies) is whether they are Medicare-certified. Certified agencies must comply with conditions of participation specified by the Centers for Medicare and Medicaid Services (CMS). Approximately 40 percent of all home health agencies are Medicare-certified.

There are three types of home health agency ownership: voluntary non-profit, government, and proprietary. Agencies can either be freestanding or components of another type of organization (such as a health system, hospital, or nursing home).

Here is a profile of home health agencies and care:

- During a typical year, seven million people (3 percent of the population) use home health services provided by about twenty thousand agencies.
- The age distribution of clients is 34 percent under sixty-five; 24 percent sixty-five to seventy-four, and 42 percent over seventy-five.
- Sixty-four percent of clients are female, 36 percent male.
- Sixty-three percent of clients are white; 8 percent are black, and the race or ethnicity of the remaining 29 percent is unspecified.
- The charge for a home health visit averages about ninety dollars.
- Of the $36 billion expended for home care annually, 40 percent is financed by Medicare, 15 percent Medicaid, 11 percent private insurance, 22 percent out-of-pocket, and 12 percent other.
- Of Medicare-certified agencies, 41 percent are freestanding proprietary and 30 percent are hospital-based.
- Eleven percent of Medicare beneficiaries use home health care during an average year (up from about 2 percent in 1974).
- The most common diagnoses of home health clients are diabetes, chronic hypertension, heart failure, arthritis, cerebrovascular disease, and chronic airway obstruction.
- Thirty-nine percent of clients have three or more conditions that restrict activities of daily living.
- Forty percent of clients live alone, 60 percent with others.

MENTAL HEALTH CARE

Mental disease encompasses an array of psychological, biological, chemical, neurological, and behavioral disorders that impair cognitive, affective, and social functioning. Some illustrations are:

- Common mental illnesses, such as depression, anxiety, and phobias
- Severe mental illness, such as psychosis, schizophrenia, and major depression
- Behavioral problems such as obsessive-compulsive disorders
- Mental retardation
- Deterioration in brain function, such as Alzheimer's disease and dementia
- Substance abuse

An estimated 40 percent of the population experience one or more psychiatric disorders requiring some form of care during their lifetime.

In the first half of the twentieth century, most common mental disorders went untreated; individuals with major problems received care in local government psychiatric hospitals. Between the mid-1950s and the early 1980s, the inpatient population decreased significantly because of the development of an array of effective psychotropic medications, expansion of ambulatory treatment alternatives, and changing societal norms regarding people with mental or behavioral disabilities.

In 1996, total mental expenditures were estimated to be $69 billion (up from $4 billion in 1969); 47 percent derived from private sources and 53 percent from the government. The source of funding by type of payer is shown in Table 2.5.

Mental health care is provided in inpatient and outpatient facilities. By far the greatest volume of services is ambulatory, offered in settings such as:

- Primary care physician offices
- Psychiatrists' offices

Table 2.5 Approximate Sources
of Funding for Mental Health Services

Source	Percentage
Public	47
Private insurance	27
Out-of-pocket	17
Other	3
Private	53
Medicaid	19
State and local government	18
Medicare	14
Federal	2

- Offices of mental health professionals (psychologists, clinical social workers, marriage and family counselors)
- Mental health centers
- General hospital outpatient departments and emergency rooms
- Day care programs
- Substance abuse centers
- Psychiatric clinics
- Focused programs such as Alcoholics Anonymous
- Support groups

Inpatient treatment is offered in psychiatric units of short-term general hospitals, mental hospitals, and special purpose hospitals (such as substance-abuse facilities). There are approximately fifty-seven hundred mental health facilities; their distribution is shown in Table 2.6.

Table 2.6. Ambulatory and Inpatient Mental Health Facilities

Facilities	Number
Total	5,722
State and county mental hospitals	229
Private psychiatric hospitals	348
Nonfederal general psychiatric services[1]	1,707
Department of Veterans Affairs[2]	145
Residential treatment facilities for emotionally disturbed children	461
Other[3]	2,832

Notes: [1]Designated psychiatric units in short-term, general hospitals

[2]Includes VA neuropsychiatric hospitals, VA general hospital psychiatric services, and VA psychiatric outpatient units

[3]Includes freestanding psychiatric outpatient clinics, partial care organizations, and multiservice mental health

HEALTH SYSTEMS

A health system combines into a single enterprise organizations that could function independently. Systems are typically defined or classified along two dimensions: the type of organizations that are combined, and the mechanism employed to do so.

As depicted in Figure 2.4, there are two primary system types: horizontal and vertical. Horizontal systems combine functionally similar organizations, such as groups of short-term general hospitals, physician practices, or nursing homes. Vertical systems combine functionally different organizations, where patient outputs of one organization in the system (a physician group practice) are inputs of another (a hospital). Horizontal systems can be composed of similar organizations in a particular market (such as a city) or those spread across a number of markets (for example, hospitals

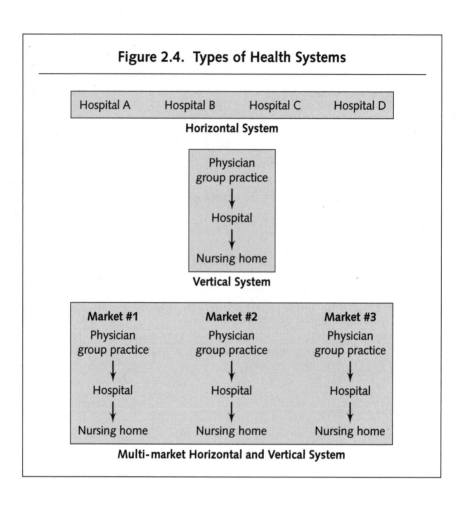

Figure 2.4. Types of Health Systems

Hospital A   Hospital B   Hospital C   Hospital D

Horizontal System

Physician group practice
↓
Hospital
↓
Nursing home

Vertical System

Market #1	Market #2	Market #3
Physician group practice	Physician group practice	Physician group practice
↓	↓	↓
Hospital	Hospital	Hospital
↓	↓	↓
Nursing home	Nursing home	Nursing home

Multi-market Horizontal and Vertical System

located in various regions of the country). Vertical systems always combine organizations within a given market. The reason is that flows of patients among combined organizations require geographic proximity. These two system types can also be combined, as with several vertical systems operating in different markets.

Systems can be formed through a variety of mechanisms (employed alone or in combination):

- Ownership—organizations built or acquired through a purchase or merger
- Affiliation—agreement among organizations to cooperate with each other
- Contracts—arrangement where one organization manages another
- Joint venture—for instance, a hospital and collection of physicians creating a health plan
- Lease—such as a hospital assuming control of a nursing home for a specified period of time

From the mid-1980s through the 1990s, the personal health care segment of the industry underwent significant consolidation. Horizontal combinations, particularly among hospitals, sought to achieve economies of scale (where fixed overhead costs were spread across organizations) and build share in local markets to increase bargaining power vis-à-vis health insurance plans. Vertical combinations were undertaken to create a continuum of services ("one-stop shopping") attractive to patients and managed care contractors.

PUBLIC HEALTH SERVICES

Whereas personal health care deals with the provision of curative services to individuals, public health focuses on the prevention of disease and promotion of health in populations.

Protection of the nation's public health is a government responsibility. In 2000, expenditures for public health were $44 billion, up from $7 billion in 1980.

Core public health functions are:

- Assessment

    Evaluating community health needs

    Investigating the occurrence of health hazards

    Analyzing the determinants of health problems

- Policy development

  Advocating and building constituencies

  Setting priorities

  Formulating plans and policies
- Assurance

  Managing resources and developing organizational infrastructure

  Implementing programs

  Evaluating program outcomes

  Informing and educating the public

These functions are performed through a complex set of relationships, as well as division of effort among federal, state, and local government public health agencies.

Federal

Federal responsibilities for public health are discharged primarily by the cabinet-level Department of Health and Human Services (DHHS). Approximately 80 percent of the department's budget is consumed by two programs: Social Security and Medicare/Medicaid.

These are the major public health functions of DHHS and corresponding agencies that perform them:

- Data gathering and analysis, and surveillance and control (National Center for Health Statistics, and Centers for Disease Control and Prevention)
- Conducting and sponsoring research (National Institute of Health)
- Providing programmatic assistance to state and local governments (Health Resources and Services Administration)
- Formulating objectives and policy (Office of the Assistant Secretary for Health)
- Ensuring the safety of food and drugs (Food and Drug Administration, and Agency for Toxic Substances and Disease Registry)

- Ensuring access to health care services by the aged and poor (Centers for Medicare and Medicaid Services)
- Providing direct services to special populations (Indian Health Service)

The nation's primary public health agency is the Centers for Disease Control and Prevention (CDC), headquartered in Atlanta. Its annual budget is approximately $3 billion, and it employs seventy-five hundred people.

State

The first state board (department) of public health was created by Massachusetts in 1855. All states and territories have departments or agencies performing public health functions, including:

- Health care professional (physician, dentist, chiropractic, pharmacist, optometrist, nursing, veterinary) licensing
- Health care facility inspection and licensing
- Vital statistics collection
- Epidemiological investigation and analysis
- Communicable disease surveillance
- Disease and tumor registration
- Laboratory services
- Policy and legislation formulation and analysis
- Health education

Local

There are approximately three thousand local public health agencies in the United States; they spend about $13 billion per year and employ about 135,000 people. Their sources of funding are local government (44 percent), state government (40 percent), federal government (3 percent), service reimbursement (billing insurance companies, Medicare and Medicaid for provision of covered personal health services, 19 percent), and other (4 percent). The distribution of local public health agencies by jurisdiction is county (60 percent), town or township (15 percent), city (10 percent), multicounty (8 percent), city-county (7 percent), and other (2 percent).

Most front-line public health services are provided locally. Examples are:

- Food safety
- Sanitation
- Sewage disposal
- Insect and pest control
- Drinking water purification
- Restaurant inspection and licensing
- Communicable disease surveillance and immunization
- Investigation of control of sexually transmitted diseases (STD)
- Public health education

Local agencies, in addition to their purely public health functions, also provide personal health services: disease screening, primary care, mental health care, maternal and child health, family planning, and in some instances hospital care (typically for the poor, through city or county hospitals). Approximately forty million people annually receive some type of personal health care from local departments of public health.

Private Initiatives

Personal health care providers (such as hospitals, nursing homes, HMOs, physicians, and clinics) play a significant role in public health. They engage in surveillance and monitoring, administer immunizations, screen for communicable diseases, and offer patient education. They cooperate with state and local departments of public health by acquiring data and coordinating the provision of personal and public health services. Many managed care organizations responsible for the care of a population of beneficiaries/members, also undertake large and sophisticated health promotion and disease prevention activities.

CHAPTER 3

Health Care Financing

ealth care is the nation's second largest industry, exceeded only by durable goods manufacturing. In 2000, total industry expenditures were $1.3 trillion, accounting for 13.2 percent of the gross domestic product (GDP), as compared with $27 billion and 5 percent of GDP in 1960 (see Figure 3.1).

The United States spends a greater percentage of its GDP on health care than any other industrialized country does; some illustrative international

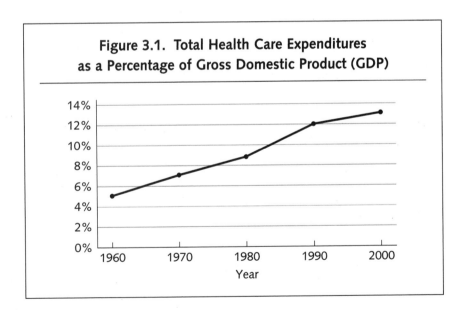

Figure 3.1. Total Health Care Expenditures as a Percentage of Gross Domestic Product (GDP)

comparisons are Germany, 10.3 percent; France, 9.4 percent; Canada, 9.3 percent; Sweden, 7.9 percent; Japan, 7.4 percent; United Kingdom, 6.9 percent; and Finland, 6.8 percent.

Figures 3.2 and 3.3 depict the source and destination of total health care expenditures.

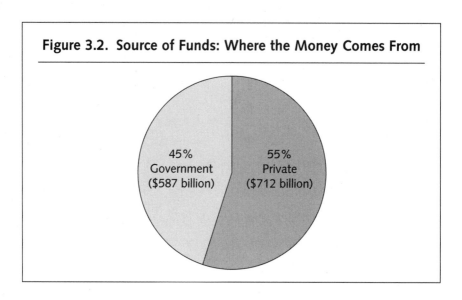

Figure 3.2. Source of Funds: Where the Money Comes From

45%
Government
($587 billion)

55%
Private
($712 billion)

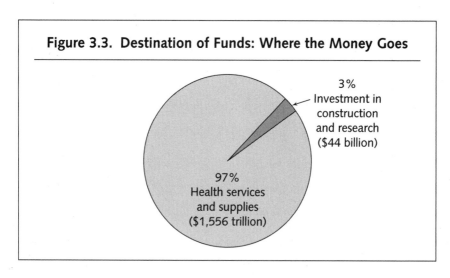

Figure 3.3. Destination of Funds: Where the Money Goes

3%
Investment in
construction
and research
($44 billion)

97%
Health services
and supplies
($1,556 trillion)

The money comes from two sources: private funds (individuals, households, and businesses); and government funds (federal, state, and local). The distribution has changed dramatically over time: in 1960, 75 percent of total expenditures came from private sources and 25 percent came from government, while in 2000 55 percent came from private funds and 45 percent from the federal government.

The $1.33 trillion spent on health care services and supplies is distributed as shown in Figure 3.4. Fully 80 percent is for hospitals, professional services (such as physicians, dentists, podiatrists, and optometrists), and retail health products (primarily pharmaceuticals). The largest components, hospital and professional services, are evenly split, about one-third of the total each.

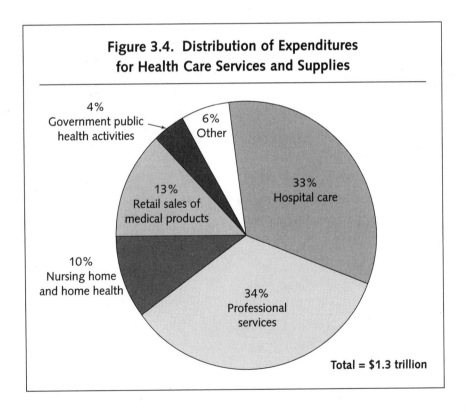

Figure 3.4. Distribution of Expenditures for Health Care Services and Supplies

CHANGING ECONOMIC DYNAMICS

The underlying "economic calculus" of health care is undergoing significant change. The most recent round began in the mid-1980s and will fundamentally reshape the industry over the next several decades. These changes, summarized in Figure 3.5, are purchaser-driven and concern who the purchasers are, what they want and expect, and how they pay.

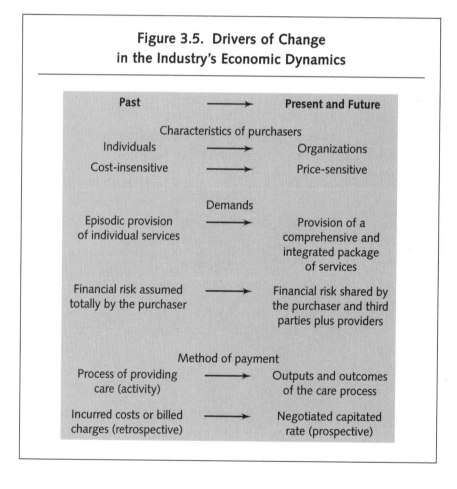

Figure 3.5. Drivers of Change in the Industry's Economic Dynamics

Past	⟶	Present and Future
Characteristics of purchasers		
Individuals	⟶	Organizations
Cost-insensitive	⟶	Price-sensitive
Demands		
Episodic provision of individual services	⟶	Provision of a comprehensive and integrated package of services
Financial risk assumed totally by the purchaser	⟶	Financial risk shared by the purchaser and third parties plus providers
Method of payment		
Process of providing care (activity)	⟶	Outputs and outcomes of the care process
Incurred costs or billed charges (retrospective)	⟶	Negotiated capitated rate (prospective)

The Way It Was

From the end of World War II through the early 1990s, individual patients sought care from physicians and hospitals for discrete episodes of illness. Patients either paid directly for this care or (increasingly) through health insurance provided by their employers—and, after 1966, with the implementation of Medicare and Medicaid, by government funding. Those with coverage were relatively price-insensitive because they bore little, or none, of the costs for services they used. Voluntary (private) and government health insurance plans paid providers full rates, either incurred costs or billed charges. More provider activity (patient days, visits, and procedures) produced greater revenues.

The Present and Future

By the late 1980s, the purchaser side of the market was dominated by large organizations (corporations and federal and state governments) who paid for health care coverage for groups of beneficiaries (employees, Medicare or Medicaid recipients).

From 1965 through the early 1990s, health care costs and expenditures increased dramatically, seriously eroding the global competitiveness of businesses and overwhelming federal, state, and local government budgets. At the same time, purchasers were beginning to question what they were getting for their money. Even though the United States had the highest per capita health care expenditures in the world, its citizens were considerably less healthy than those in most other industrialized countries. Pressure for making significant changes in the nation's health care system increased.

Being eaten alive by increasing costs, businesses and government became increasingly price-sensitive. They wanted to predict and control their expenditures for health care and shift some of the financial risk to health insurers and providers. For a set price, they demanded a comprehensive or integrated package of services where providers were paid set rates per beneficiary, irrespective of the costs they incurred.

FLOW OF FUNDS THROUGH THE SYSTEM

Expenditures for personal health care services and products include institutional services (for example, hospital and nursing home care), professional services (from physicians, dentists, podiatrists, chiropractors), products (durable medical equipment and so on), and supplies (notably, pharmaceuticals). In 1960, $23 billion was spent on personal health care services ($126 per person); 1999 expenditures were $1.068 trillion ($3,808 per person). Over the past four decades, such expenditures have increased in absolute dollars by a factor of forty-six and per capita thirtyfold.

Over the period 1960–2000, expenditures for personal health care grew about 10 percent each year (see Figure 3.6). The causes of this increase were:

- *Economywide,* stemming from inflation in the economy as a whole
- *Medical,* inflation in the medical component of the consumer price index

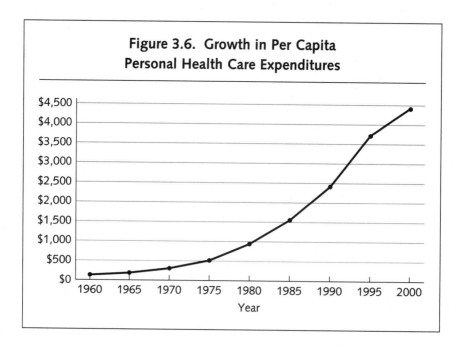

Figure 3.6. Growth in Per Capita Personal Health Care Expenditures

- *Population,* overall growth in the population
- *Intensity,* changes in the type and quality of health care services provided

The relative contribution of each factor to the overall increase in health care costs is noted in Figure 3.7.

Figure 3.8 depicts the flow of personal health care expenditures through the industry. Expenditures come from three sources: (1) households (individuals and families) who purchase health insurance, pay portions of premiums (to supplement contributions by employers and government), make coinsurance and deductible payments, and purchase health care services directly; (2) employers who purchase health insurance coverage for their employees; and (3) federal, state, and local governments that pay for all or a portion of coverage for certain designated populations (for instance, the aged and poor) in addition to providing services directly (as through public, Veterans Administration, and military hospitals and clinics). Typically, expenditures by individuals and employers purchase health insurance coverage. Payments are made through a variety of mechanisms

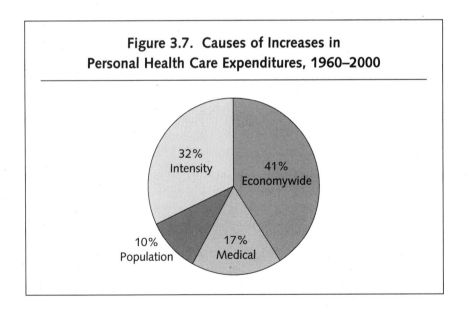

Figure 3.7. Causes of Increases in Personal Health Care Expenditures, 1960–2000

32% Intensity

41% Economywide

10% Population

17% Medical

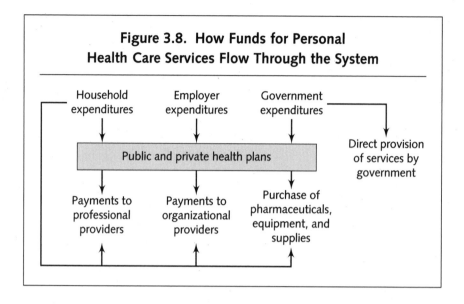

Figure 3.8. How Funds for Personal Health Care Services Flow Through the System

Household expenditures →
Employer expenditures →
Government expenditures →

Public and private health plans

Direct provision of services by government

Payments to professional providers

Payments to organizational providers

Purchase of pharmaceuticals, equipment, and supplies

(which are described in the next section) to professionals and organizations in addition to paying for drugs, medical supplies, and equipment.

Data on expenditures and receipt of funds are not precisely captured employing these categories, but Table 3.1 offers some rough estimates based on the most recent available data (drawn from various sources).

HEALTH INSURANCE

Health insurance is an umbrella term used to describe a variety of methods for financing the provision of health care services.

Insurance spreads the risk of financial loss associated with an event among members of a group. Traditionally, it is provided (underwritten) in those instances where the potential loss is large (catastrophic) and beyond the ability of a group member to pay in the short run; has a monetary value; cannot be influenced or controlled by a group member; and is predictable for the group as a whole over a specified period of time.

Table 3.1. Estimates of Funds Flow for Personal Health Care Services

Category	Amount (in Billions)	Percentage of Category
Expenditures for personal health care	$866	100
Household[1]	$323	37
Employers[2]	$250	29
Government[3]	$203	23
Other	$90	11
Direct provision of services by federal, state, and local governments[4]	$158	100
Total receipts for provision of personal health care services	$866	100
Organizations[5]	$449	52
Professionals[6]	$317	37
Pharmaceuticals, supplies, and equipment	$101	11

Notes: [1]Includes individual out-of-pocket payments for the direct purchase of services; purchase of individual health insurance policies (primary and supplemental); employee premiums for employment-based health insurance; deductible and coinsurance payments; balance billings; and premiums paid for Medicare Part B coverage.

[2]Includes contributions to health insurance premiums; contributions to Medicare; and workers' compensation payments.

[3]Includes contributions to private health insurance premiums, and Medicaid.

[4]For example, Department of Veterans Affairs, U.S. military, Indian Health Service, and state and local public hospitals.

[5]For example, hospitals, nursing homes, home health agencies, and hospices.

[6]For example, physicians, dentists, chiropractors, podiatrists, and optometrists.

The risks and losses associated with the use of most personal health care services do not meet these criteria. For example, routine health care expenditures for an individual or family are small, discretionary, and predictable. Accordingly, health insurance is not pure insurance, but rather a form of prepayment where small periodic outlays are made on the basis of the likelihood of expenditures by members of a group. Bowing to convention, the term *health insurance* is used here.

There are three basic types of health insurance:

- *Voluntary health insurance,* bought by individuals and purchased by employers for their employees or retirees from nonprofit and commercial health plans (Blue Cross, Aetna, Cigna, and others)
- *Social insurance,* provided by a government health plan as a benefit that is earned (for instance, Medicare)
- *Public welfare insurance,* provided by government to eligible individuals on the basis of need (Medicaid)

Approximately 84 percent of the population is covered by some form of health insurance, although benefits vary widely. The number of enrollees and their distribution are shown in Table 3.2.

In 2000, forty-one million persons, 17 percent of the population below age sixty-five, had no health insurance coverage—an increase from thirty-two million uninsured and 15 percent of the nonelderly population in 1987

Table 3.2. Health Insurance Coverage

	Number of Enrollees (Millions)	Percentage of Population Covered
Private	171	63
Medicare	39	16
Medicaid	24	9

(see Figure 3.9). During this period, the number of uninsured increased by more than one-third. The Census Bureau estimates that those without health insurance will grow to fifty-three to sixty million by 2007, 21 to 25 percent of the nonelderly population.

The growth in the uninsured over the past decade is due to three factors:

- An increase in health care costs relative to average family income, thus making insurance less affordable.

- An increase in the absolute number of families living at or below the federally specified poverty level. These individuals account for 30 percent of the uninsured, and Medicaid covers only about 50 percent of them.

- A decrease in the number of firms that provide health insurance for their employees. Fully 65 percent of the uninsured live in families

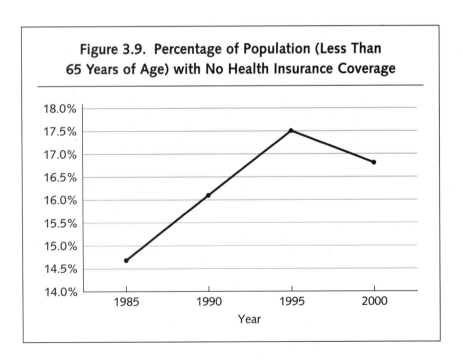

Figure 3.9. Percentage of Population (Less Than 65 Years of Age) with No Health Insurance Coverage

headed by a full-time, full-year worker. The percentage of the non-elderly population with employment-linked health insurance decreased from 69 percent in 1987 to 64 percent in 1997.

Lack of health insurance coverage varies considerably by state. Those with the highest percentage of uninsured are Arizona (26 percent), New Mexico (25 percent), Texas (24 percent), Oklahoma (22 percent), Louisiana (22 percent), and Florida (21 percent). States with the lowest percentage of their population without any type of health insurance coverage are Rhode Island (7 percent), New Hampshire (8 percent), Pennsylvania (9 percent), Connecticut (10 percent), and Minnesota (11 percent).

Uninsured rates are affected by a number of sociodemographic and economic characteristics; illustrations are presented in Table 3.3.

TYPES OF HEALTH INSURANCE PLANS

All health insurance involves a contractual relationship among four parties:

1. *Purchasers,* the primary payer (typically employers and federal, state, and local governments)

2. *Beneficiaries,* the users of health care services

3. *Health plans,* organizations that collect premiums, reimburse providers, and perform other administrative functions

4. *Providers,* organizations and individual professionals who deliver health care services

The three basic types of health insurance plans (indemnity, service benefit, and managed care) are defined by the contractual relationships among these parties.

Indemnity Plan

In the most typical arrangement, there is a contract between a beneficiary and a health plan. The beneficiary pays a premium to the health plan (sometimes in addition to a contribution made by that person's employer).

Table 3.3. Sociodemographic and Economic Factors Affecting Insurance Coverage

	Percentage of Population (Less Than Age 65) Uninsured
Age	
Under 18	12
18–44	22
45–64	13
Gender	
Male	18
Female	18
Race and ethnicity	
White	15
Black	20
Hispanic	35
Poverty level[1]	
Below 100 percent	34
100–149 percent	37
150–199 percent	27
200 percent and above	9
Residence[2]	
Within an MSA	16
Outside an MSA	19

Notes: [1]The poverty level is established by the federal government on the basis of a number of factors (family size, annual income, and so on). Below 100 percent (the specified poverty level) is considered poor.

[2]Metropolitan statistical areas (MSAs) are urban regions designated by the Census Bureau.

When a covered service is used, the health plan reimburses the beneficiary, who then pays the provider.

The key features of this type of plan (as depicted in Figure 3.10) are that there is no contractual relationship between the health plan and providers, the payment by a health plan to the beneficiary is a set dollar amount for a specific service (for example, $400 for each day of hospital stay, or $40 per physician office visit) irrespective of the provider's charge, and the beneficiary is responsible for paying the provider directly.

Service Benefit Plan

The most common arrangement is the one seen in Figure 3.11. Typically, a purchaser (employer) contracts with a health plan and pays it a premium for each beneficiary (employee and family members); beneficiaries usually make contributions that cover a portion of the premium. The health plan contracts with provider hospitals or professionals to offer a specific array

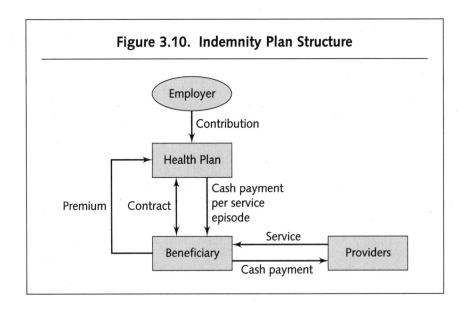

Figure 3.10. Indemnity Plan Structure

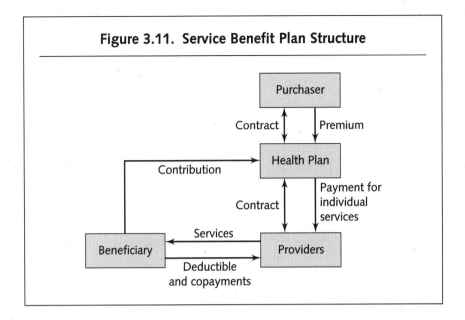

Figure 3.11. Service Benefit Plan Structure

of services to beneficiaries for a negotiated payment (cost, charges, discounted charges, or set rate). Beneficiaries usually make deductible and coinsurance payments to providers when they receive service, but they are not liable for any other charges associated with covered benefits.

The key features of this type of plan are that payments are made to providers by the health plan on behalf of beneficiaries for covered services, and beneficiaries receive services rather than cash payments (as in an indemnity plan).

Managed Care Plan

Managed care is a special type of service benefit plan that combines health insurance and provider functions (see Figure 3.12).

The purchaser contracts with a health plan for a package of services on behalf of a beneficiary group for which it pays a set amount per enrollee per month. The health plan has a contractual (and occasionally, ownership)

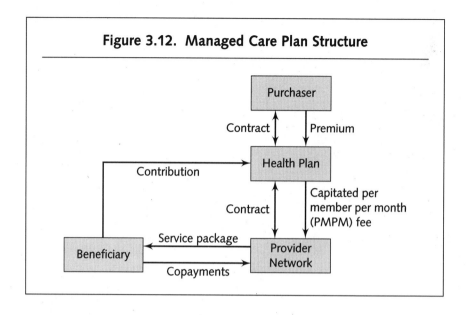

Figure 3.12. Managed Care Plan Structure

relationship with a network of providers to whom it pays a fixed rate per member per month to provide covered services. Beneficiaries are often responsible for a copayment at the point of service, but not a deductible. Additionally, beneficiaries are subject to restrictions regarding choice of provider. Other than for the provision of emergency services, they must use providers within the health plan's network. When using out-of-network providers, they incur larger copayments or may have no coverage.

The distinctive features of a managed care plan are that a comprehensive and integrated service package (rather than individual services) is provided to beneficiaries; and the health plan's contract is with a network of organizations and professionals to provide all covered services for a fixed payment, regardless of utilization and costs. As a consequence, the health plan and/or provider network bears the financial risk associated with all covered care for a designated population over a period of time.

There are numerous variations on these three basic health plan types.

VOLUNTARY HEALTH INSURANCE

Voluntary health insurance (VHI) is a diverse array of mechanisms for financing health care services obtained through private (nonprofit and commercial) sources; it is offered by businesses as an employee benefit or purchased directly by individuals. VHI can serve as the sole source of coverage or it can supplement benefits provided by social health insurance, such as Medicare (addressed in the next section).

The first VHI plan (providing indemnity payments for loss of income due to illness and injury) was offered by Franklin Health Insurance in the 1850s. The number of health insurance companies grew slowly during the late nineteenth and early twentieth centuries. Contemporary VHI can be dated to 1929, when Baylor Hospital in Dallas insured a group of public school teachers for inpatient hospital expenses; this was the first Blue Cross Plan. Other similar plans were created in the early 1930s. In 1939, the California Medical Society offered a VHI plan to cover in-hospital physician services; this was the first Blue Shield Plan. During the 1940s and 1950s, many of these plans merged their operations (typically in individual states) and were represented, at the national level, by the Blue Cross and Blue Shield Association.

As noted in Figure 3.13, 72 percent of the population has some form of VHI; of those with such coverage, fully 88 percent is provided through their place of employment.

There are four basic types of VHI plan: commercial, the "Blues," HMOs, and self-funded.

- *Commercial* plans can be either nonprofit or for-profit; some are mutuals (owned by their policy holders), others are stock corporations.
- *Blue Cross and/or Blue Shield* plans are closely tied to the hospital industry and medical profession, often operate under special state-enabling laws, and are generally not subject to the same regulations as commercial plans. Blues were the first to offer service rather than indemnity benefits on the basis of communitywide ratings (which charge everyone the same

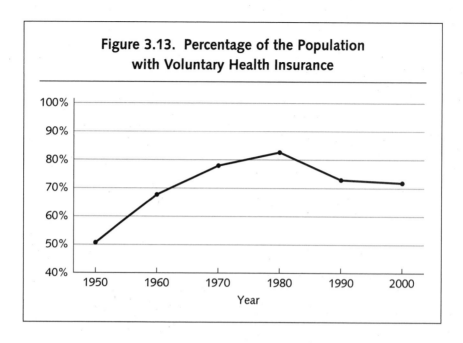

Figure 3.13. Percentage of the Population with Voluntary Health Insurance

premium regardless of their characteristics). Historically, they have been nonprofit entities; however, in recent years some have converted to for-profit status and many have commercial subsidiaries.

- *HMOs,* or health maintenance organizations (addressed in a subsequent section), combine underwriting (the insurance function) with delivery of health services through an owned or contracted network of providers.

- *Self-funded* plans are typically sponsored by employers, who bear the full financial risk of providing health care benefits to employees, dependents, and retirees. They do not purchase insurance from, or pay premiums to, a health plan, although they may contract with an insurance company (commercial, Blue, or other entity) to provide administrative services.

VHI enrollment is split roughly in thirds among commercial, Blue, and HMO Plus self-funded plans.

The nature of VHI coverage varies by:

- *Benefit type,* which can either be indemnity or service
- *Contribution,* a proportion of the total premium paid by beneficiaries (versus that contributed by others, such as an employer)
- *Coverage,* type of benefits provided (hospital care, physician services, drugs, vision care) and their comprehensiveness or inclusiveness (for example, number of routine physician office visits per year)
- *Deductible and co-insurance rates,* amount of expenditures that must be borne by the beneficiary before plan payments "kick in," and the proportion of fees paid by beneficiaries for each service
- *Exclusions and limitations,* such as waiting periods (for example, a certain number of months of employment before the plan becomes active), and coverage of preexisting conditions

VHI coverage is generally dependent upon, and linked to, employment. Approximately 50 percent of private sector establishments (employing about 80 percent of the nongovernmental workforce) offer VHI to their employees.

SOCIAL HEALTH INSURANCE (MEDICARE)

Medicare is the health care industry's largest payer. In 2000, it covered forty million people (14 percent of the population) and expended $227 billion (about $5,500 per enrollee); $88 billion in Medicare funding went to hospitals, making up about 30 percent of their total patient revenues; and $37 billion went to physicians, accounting for about 20 percent of their total revenues.

Medicare was enacted in 1965 as an amendment (Title 18) to the Social Security Act. It is a federally sponsored program that provides health insurance to individuals over sixty-five years of age in addition to disabled persons receiving Social Security benefits and those with end-stage renal disease. Medicare is not welfare; individuals make contributions to the program through payroll deductions and are entitled to receive benefits. The program is managed by the Centers for Medicare and Medicaid Services.

Medicare is actually two separate, although coordinated, programs: *Part A,* a compulsory health plan that covers hospital-based services; and *Part B,* a voluntary, supplemental health plan that covers professional (primarily physician) services.

Part A

Financing: Part A hospital insurance is funded by a payroll tax paid into the Social Security (Medicare) Trust Fund. Employees contribute 1.45 percent of wages, matched equally by employers; self-employed individuals pay 2.9 percent of earnings.

Benefits: the program provides ninety days of inpatient hospital care per episode of illness, a life-time reserve of sixty days of inpatient hospital care that can be drawn upon when the maximum for an episode of illness is exceeded, and home health visits following an inpatient admission.

Payments: for each episode of illness, beneficiaries pay a deductible equal to the charge for one day of hospital care. A copayment is made for each of the sixty-first through ninetieth days of inpatient hospital care equal to 25 percent of the deductible.

Provider reimbursement: from the inception of the program until 1983, hospitals were reimbursed for their costs of providing care as defined by a complex set of regulations and formulas. Hospitals received estimated monthly payments, which were adjusted at year end on the basis of a cost report submitted to the Health Care Financing Administration (now the Centers for Medicare and Medicaid Services). Beginning in 1983, Medicare switched to a prospective payment system. A payment rate is assigned to five hundred diagnosis-related groups (DRGs), on the basis of the patient's age, sex, principal and secondary diagnosis, procedure performed (if any), and discharge status. Certain costs, such as medical education and depreciation, are excluded from the DRG rate and reimbursed separately. Additionally, some hospitals (such as psychiatric, children's, rehabilitation, and long-term care) are excluded from the prospective payment system and reimbursed under different arrangements.

Part B

Financing: Part B is financed 24 percent from premiums paid by enrollees and 76 percent from federal treasury funds. The monthly premium in 2002 was $54 per month, deducted directly from an enrollee's Social Security check.

Benefits: coverage includes physician care; physician-ordered supplies, durable medical equipment, and services provided by some other categories of health professionals; and outpatient hospital care.

Provider reimbursement: prior to 1992 physicians were paid fee-for-service on the basis of their "reasonable and customary" charges. In 1992, Medicare began making payments according to a resource-based relative value scale (RBRVS). Using this system, an index number is assigned to every physician encounter or procedure according to the amount of work required to perform it, in addition to practice expenses and malpractice insurance costs. To determine payment, the index number is multiplied by a standard conversion factor (or "going rate"), which is established each year. As an illustration, for a particular surgical procedure the index number is 15, the conversion factor is $40, and the fee is 15 times $40, or $600.

WELFARE INSURANCE (MEDICAID)

Medicaid was enacted in 1965 as Title 19 of the Social Security Act. The program finances the provision of health care services to the poor. In a strict sense, Medicaid is not health insurance; rather, it is a welfare subsidy. Benefits are not earned but provided to recipients in need. The scope of Medicaid coverage is portrayed in Table 3.4.

In 2000, Medicaid covered forty-one million individuals. It is federally sponsored and supported (overseen by the Centers for Medicare and Medicaid Services) but state-administered. Fifty-seven percent of its funding is federal, and the remainder comes from the states.

Table 3.4. Medicaid at a Glance
(Percentage of Individuals Covered Under Age 65)

Attribute	Percentage
Total covered under the age of 65	9
Age	
Under 6	24
6—17	17
18—44	6
45—64	5
Gender	
Male	8
Female	11
Race	
White	7
Black	19
Hispanic	14
Poverty level*	
Below 100 percent	37
100—149 percent	20
150—199 percent	11
200 percent or greater	2

Note: *Determined by U.S. Census Bureau criteria, including family income; family size; number of children in the family; and, for families with two or fewer adults, their age. The poverty level is set at 100 percent; thus, for example, 200 percent is an income of twice the poverty level.

States choose whether to have a Medicaid program; all but Arizona have decided to do so. Each state determines the financial, need-based criteria that individuals must meet to be enrolled. Federal law mandates the provision of certain minimum benefits, such as physician services; nonpreventive dental services; hospital inpatient care; hospital outpatient care; nursing home care; home health visits, and laboratory and X-ray services. Optional benefits can be included at a state's discretion: inpatient psychiatric care, optometrist care and eyeglasses, routine dental care, and prescription drugs. States determine utilization limits for both mandated and optional benefits and establish eligibility criteria, in addition to specifying the methods and rates for paying providers.

HEALTH MAINTENANCE ORGANIZATIONS

An HMO is a hybrid health care insurance and provider mechanism that offers a type of managed care plan. In its simplest form, an HMO links together (through contracts or ownership) in one entity a health plan, hospitals, and physicians.

The key components and their relationships (depicted in Figure 3.14) are:

- A *health plan,* which contracts with purchasers, underwrites the financial risk of providing care, negotiates and manages relationships with providers, pays providers, and performs administrative functions.
- *Hospitals,* which provide inpatient health care services to beneficiaries and may include other entities such as nursing home, home health, rehabilitation, and mental or behavioral health facilities.
- *Physicians,* who provide primary and specialty medical services to beneficiaries and may include other professionals such as chiropractors, podiatrists, and psychologists.

In *relationship A,* the health plan can either contract with or own organizational providers; the former type of relationship is far more common than the latter. In *relationship B,* the health plan can secure professional services in three ways:

1. Contract with individual physicians, who remain independent and care for beneficiaries, in addition to other patients, in their offices (called an IPA, or independent practice association, model HMO)

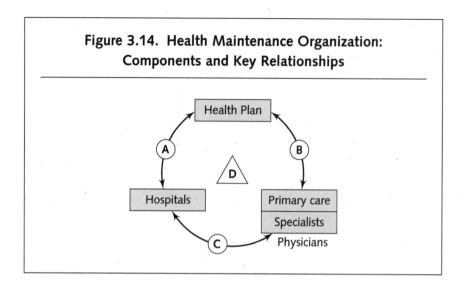

Figure 3.14. Health Maintenance Organization: Components and Key Relationships

2. Contract with organized groups of physicians, who either care for plan beneficiaries exclusively or do so in addition to other patients (called a group model HMO)

3. Hire physicians as employees (called a staff model HMO)

In *relationship C,* health plan hospitals can be either closed-staff or open-staff. In a closed arrangement, only physicians who are employees of, or have contracted with, the health plan are medical staff members. In an open arrangement, health plan and other physicians are admitted to the medical staff.

Relationship D is the essential glue that binds the three parties together and structures their relationships with purchasers and beneficiaries. It consists of administration arrangements and economic incentives designed to increase clinical quality and efficiency, manage utilization of services, and control costs:

- Limiting the type of benefits and services available to those deemed clinically and cost-effective

- Restrictions on use of nonplan providers

- Payment of set rates to hospitals and physicians (per beneficiary per month) for providing covered services irrespective of their amount and cost
- Provision of health promotion and disease prevention services
- Utilization of primary care physicians as gatekeepers who manage patients' use of hospital and specialist care
- Authorization of services before they are provided
- Employment of clinical protocols and pathways to manage a patient's total episode of illness
- Utilization and quality monitoring and review

There are a number of variations on this basic structure:

- An HMO can be either an independent organization or a component of a health plan (like Blue Cross).
- HMOs can be either nonprofit or for-profit and owned or controlled by a separate corporation, hospital, or physician group.
- An HMO can own the health plan and hospitals but contract with independent medical groups to provide professional services. For example, in each of the regions in which it operates, Kaiser Foundation Health Plan (which operates its own hospitals) contracts with Kaiser Permanente Medical Group (an independent professional corporation).
- An HMO may employ primary care physicians and contract to provide specialty care.
- An HMO might own its hospitals and contract with a medical group but also have contracts with nonowned hospitals and independent physicians to provide some subspecialty services (for instance, cardiac surgery and transplants).

In 2000, approximately eighty-one million Americans, or 30 percent of the population, received their health care through an HMO. Growth in the number of HMO enrollees and percent of the population covered by them are shown in Figures 3.15 and 3.16.

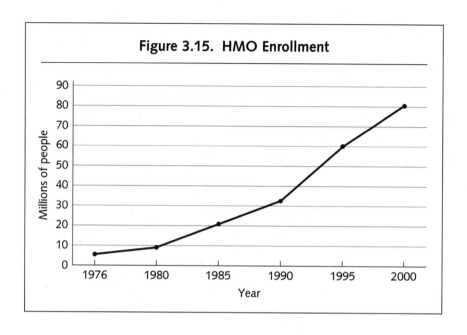

Figure 3.15. HMO Enrollment

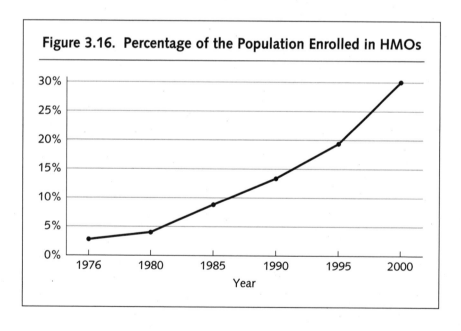

Figure 3.16. Percentage of the Population Enrolled in HMOs

In 2000, there were 568 HMOs, up from 174 in 1976, a 226 percent increase over the period. The types of plans, in terms of their relationships with physicians, are shown in Table 3.5.

Table 3.5. Types of HMO Plans		
Type	**Number of Plans**	**Percentage of Total HMO Enrollment**
IPA[1]	257	42
Group[2]	104	20
Mixed[3]	180	38

Notes: [1]Professional services provided by contract independent medical groups and individual physicians (who continue to see non-HMO patients).

[2]Professional services provided by employed physicians and/or exclusively contracted groups.

[3]Combination of IPA and group models.

CHAPTER 4

Health Care Personnel

The health care industry is one of the nation's largest employers (see Figure 4.1).

Nearly twelve million individuals hold jobs in health care (91 percent in the private sector and 9 percent in government); this comprises a little over 8 percent of the civilian workforce, up from 1.5 percent in 1920 and 3 percent in 1960. Employment is expected to increase 25 percent by 2010, as compared with 16 percent for the economy as a whole. Health care will account for 13 percent of all new jobs created between 2000 and 2010; nine of the top twenty occupations projected to be the economy's fastest growing over this period will be in health care.

A distinction is typically made between professions and occupations. Members of a profession are responsible for performing critical and highly complex tasks; undergo a lengthy education process; master a large body of knowledge upon which their practice is based; have a direct relationship with clients and serve as their agents; exercise a high level of autonomy and discretion regarding the nature of their practice and the context in which it occurs; control (with minimal outside influence) entry into, and preparation for, the profession; and are licensed or credentialed. The difference between professions and occupations is a continuum, not a dichotomy. The prototypical profession, against which all others are compared, is medicine.

The health care workforce is composed of 45 percent professional and related occupations (such as physicians, nurses, pharmacists, and other direct care givers), 30 percent service workers (patient assistants, attendants,

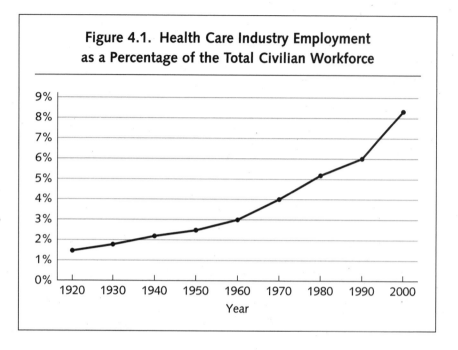

Figure 4.1. Health Care Industry Employment as a Percentage of the Total Civilian Workforce

and aides; food preparation, maintenance and housekeeping), 18 percent office and administrative support personnel, 5 percent managers, and 2 percent other. Part-time employees are 15 percent of the workforce. Employment by type of organization is shown in Table 4.1.

Health professionals, who provide direct patient care, are a central and critical component of the industry's workforce. Their distribution is shown in Table 4.2.

PHYSICIANS

Physicians diagnose and treat—through both medical and surgical means—illnesses and conditions that impair human functioning, and they supervise patient interactions with other health care professionals.

There are approximately 814,000 licensed physicians in the United States, about 84 percent of whom are professionally active. The number of practicing

Table 4.1. Health Care Employment by Type of Organization

Type	Number of Employees	Percentage of Total Industry Employment
Hospitals	5,189,000	43
Nursing and personal care facilities	1,745,000	15
Physician offices and clinics	1,774,000	15
Dentist offices and clinics	668,000	6
Other	2,541,000	21

Table 4.2. Distribution of Health Care Professionals

	Number (Active)	Personnel per 100,000 Population	Percentage of Total
Total	3,902,000		100
Chiropractors	49,600	18	1
Dentists	168,000	59	4
Dieticians and nutritionists	97,000	26	3
Occupational therapists	55,000	17	1
Optometrists	29,500	11	0.7
Pharmacists	208,000	69	6
Physical therapists	144,000	40	4
Physicians	772,000	266	19
Podiatrists	11,300	4	0.3
Registered nurses	2,271,000	823	58
Speech therapists	97,000	36	3

physicians has increased by a factor of 3.5 since 1950; the number of active physicians per 100,000 population has grown from 135 in 1950 to 258 in 2000 (see Figure 4.2).

There are two types of physicians: M.D.s (allopathic) and D.O.s (osteopathic). Their education and competencies are roughly equivalent. Although both M.D.s and D.O.s employ the full range of accepted diagnostic and treatment regimens (including prescribing drugs and doing surgery), osteopathic physicians typically place greater emphasis on the musculoskeletal system, preventive medicine, and holistic care. About 5 percent of active physicians are D.O.s.

A breakdown of physicians by type of practice is shown in Table 4.3. The average physician works about fifty-five hours per week and has an annual net income (after expenses) of roughly $200,000.

The geographic distribution of practicing physicians is quite uneven. States (and district) with the highest number of physicians per 100,000 population are the District of Columbia (601), Massachusetts (342), New York (329), Maryland (310), Connecticut (307), and Rhode Island (293). States

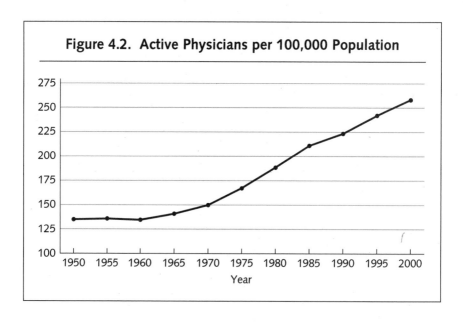

Figure 4.2. Active Physicians per 100,000 Population

The Health Care Industry: A Primer

Table 4.3. Physicians by Type of Practice

	Number	Percentage of Total Physicians
Total	813,800	100
Nonfederal	673,000	83
Involved in patient care	631,400	78
Office-based practice	490,400	60
Hospital-based practice	141,000	17
Other professional activity	41,600	5
Federal	19,400	2
Involved in patient care	16,000	2
Other	3,400	0.4
Inactive	75,200	9
Not classified	45,100	6
Unknown	2,000	0.1

with the lowest ratios are Idaho (144), Mississippi (149), Oklahoma (150), Iowa (154), and Wyoming (156). Differences in physician-population ratio are even greater across cities and between metropolitan and rural areas.

Physicians typically complete eleven to sixteen years of post–high school education, including four years as undergraduates, four years of medical school, and three to eight years of specialty (residency) and subspecialty (fellowship) training.

The four years of medical school (referred to as undergraduate medical education) is divided into a pair of two-year blocks. The first two (pre-clinical) years are spent studying basic sciences foundational to medical practice (anatomy, physiology, biochemistry, pathology, microbiology, pharmacology) and learning how to take patient histories and conduct basic physical examinations. The second two (clinical) years of training take place in patient care settings (hospitals and ambulatory care facilities) under the supervision of physician faculty members. Students learn to diagnose and treat patients and perform medical procedures by rotating through various clinical services: internal medicine, general surgery, obstetrics and gynecology, pediatrics, psychiatry, and family practice. Upon graduation, students are awarded an M.D. (doctor of medicine) or D.O. (doctor of osteopathy) degree. After completing an examination and one year of postgraduate training, they are licensed by the states.

There are 144 U.S. medical schools, of which 125 are allopathic (M.D. degree granting) and 19 osteopathic (D.O. degree granting); total enrollment is about 76,000 students. Their application-to-admission ratio is 2.6:1. Combined annual admissions are 19,500 students; 86 percent are enrolled in allopathic schools and the remainder percent in osteopathic schools. Selected student characteristics are shown in Table 4.4.

Upon completing medical school, virtually all physicians undertake specialty training (referred to as graduate medical education). Approximately 95 percent of physicians are involved in some type of specialty practice. There are eight thousand residency programs, offered by seven hundred hospitals enrolling ninety-eight thousand residents. Twenty-four percent of all residents are graduates of non-U.S. medical schools, up from 14 percent in 1990.

Table 4.4. Medical Student (M.D. Schools) Characteristics

	Percentage of Total Enrollment
Race/ethnicity	
White	64
Asian	20
Black	8
Hispanic	7
American Indian	1
Gender	
Male	56
Female	44

Residencies include some didactic instruction, but most of the training entails caring for patients under the supervision of experienced physician specialists. After completing a residency, a physician is "board-eligible." Once he or she has gained experience in treating specific types of cases and passes a written and/or oral examination, the physician becomes "board-certified." Some physicians seek additional training in fellowships leading to subspecialty certification.

There are twenty-four officially recognized medical specialties; they are listed and briefly described in Appendix B.

The distribution of nonfederal physicians involved in office-based practice across medical specialties is presented in Table 4.5.

NURSES

Comprising approximately 20 percent of the industry's workforce, nursing is the largest health care profession.

Defined by state licensing laws and shaped by the setting in which they practice, registered nurses (R.N.s) perform a broad array of tasks, including serving as patient advocates; observing, assessing, and recording symptoms in addition to progress and response to treatments; developing and undertaking nursing care plans; assisting physicians in examining and treating patients; administering medications and performing certain procedures; supervising other personnel; and educating patients and their families about follow-up care.

R.N.s are educated in three ways:

- Associate degree in nursing (A.D.N.) programs, offered by community colleges, two years in length

- Diploma programs, offered by hospital-based schools of nursing, three years in length (a degree is not awarded but undergraduate credit is often earned)

- Bachelor of science in nursing (B.S.N.) programs, offered by colleges and universities, four years in length

The distribution of registered nursing programs by type is shown in Table 4.6.

Table 4.5. Distribution of Physician Specialists

	Percentage of Total
Anesthesiology	7
Dermatology	2
Emergency medicine	3
Family practice	14
Gastroenterology	3
Internal medicine	18
Neurology	2
Obstetrics and gynecology	7
Ophthalmology	3
Orthopedic surgery	3
Otolaryngology	2
Pathology	2
Pediatrics	9
Plastic surgery	1
Psychiatry	5
Pulmonology	1
Radiology	4
Surgery (general)	5
Urology	2
Other	7

There are approximately 120,000 first-year nursing students, distributed as follows: associate degree programs, 61 percent; baccalaureate programs, 34 percent; and diploma programs, 5 percent. There has been a significant shift in graduations from nursing programs over the last twenty years. In 1980, 63 percent of R.N.s were products of diploma programs; 37 percent were A.D.N. and B.S.N. graduates. By 2000, the figures had reversed; 30 percent of registered nurses received their training in diploma programs and 70 percent were A.D.N. or B.S.N. graduates.

**Table 4.6. Distribution of
Registered Nursing Programs, by Type**

	Number	Percentage of Total
Total	1,508	100
A.D.N. programs	876	58
Diploma programs	109	7
B.S.N. programs	523	35

Nursing education consists of classroom instruction (in the biomedical and social-behavioral sciences) and supervised clinical experience in inpatient, ambulatory, and community settings. The breadth and depth of exposure and experience vary by type of program. All graduates, irrespective of program completed, are eligible to take the same national exam and receive identical licenses to practice granted by the states.

There are approximately 2,700,000 registered nurses; 59 percent work full-time, 23 percent work part-time, and 18 percent are not professionally active. The number of employed R.N.s increased from 541 per one hundred thousand in 1980 to 816 per hundred thousand in 2000. Here are selected facts regarding the nursing workforce:

- R.N.s are, on average, forty-five years old. In 1980, 53 percent of nurses were under the age of forty; in 2000, the figure was 32 percent.
- Nursing is a female-dominated profession; 94 percent of nurses are women. Seventy-two percent are married, and 53 percent have children living at home.
- Eighty-six percent of registered nurses are white, 5 percent are black, and about 4 percent are Hispanic.

The distribution of nurses by practice setting is presented in Table 4.7.

Table 4.7. Distribution of Registered Nurses, by Practice Setting

	Percentage of Employed Nurses
Hospitals	59
Public and community health organizations	18
Ambulatory care	10
Nursing homes and extended care facilities	7
Nursing education	2
Other	4

Registered nurse median annual income is $45,000. Between 1980 and 2000, salaries grew by 34 percent, not adjusted for inflation.

Approximately 7 percent of all nurses engage in some form of advanced practice (nurse practitioner, clinical nurse specialist, nurse midwife, or nurse anesthetist).

ANCILLARY NURSING PERSONNEL

The largest health care occupation is licensed practical nursing (L.P.N.s), called licensed vocational nurses (L.V.N.s) in California and Texas. L.P.N.s provide basic, nonprofessional, nursing care. They observe patients, take vital signs, keep records, and change dressings, besides assisting patients with personal hygiene, ambulation, and eating and bathing; in some states they can administer certain medications.

Training takes twelve to fourteen months in programs offered by community colleges and technical or trade schools, of which there are eleven hundred in the United States. All states require individuals to possess a high school diploma (or equivalent) and pass a licensing exam.

There are approximately seven hundred thousand employed L.P.N.s. Twenty-nine percent work in nursing homes, 28 percent in hospitals, and 14 percent in doctors' offices and other ambulatory care settings; the remainder are employed in residential care facilities and home health care agencies. The median annual income of an L.P.N. is $29,000.

DENTISTS

Dentists prevent, diagnose, and treat diseases of the mouth, teeth, gums, and associated structures.

Dental education entails four years of postbaccalaureate degree work. The first two (preclinical) years focus on the basic sciences, such as dental anatomy, physiology, microbiology, and pathology. During the second two (clinical) years, students treat patients in teaching clinics under the supervision of faculty. Graduation leads to award of a D.D.S. (doctor of dental surgery) or D.M.D. (doctor of dental medicine) degree. There are fifty-five dental schools with a total enrollment of about seventeen thousand students.

Graduates must pass a written and practical National Board Dental Examination before being granted a license to practice by the states. With an additional two to four years of postgraduate education, dentists can specialize in any of nine areas: orthodontics (straightening teeth and correcting misalignment); oral and maxiofacial surgery (operating on the mouth and jaw); pediatric dentistry (practice focused on children); periodontics (treating gums and bones supporting the teeth); prosthodontics (replacement of missing teeth); endodontics (performing root canals); public health dentistry (dental health promotion and disease prevention); oral pathology (studying dental disease); and oral and maxiofacial radiology (diagnosing diseases of the mouth, head, and neck using imaging technology).

There are 168,000 practicing dentists, 92 percent of whom are in private practice. Eighty percent of active dentists are in solo practice, and 12 percent belong to a group. Seventy-one percent of active dentists are male, 29 percent female. Their average income is $129,000.

Some dentists (particularly specialists) are granted membership on a hospital medical staff; many work in institutional settings, including nursing homes and ambulatory care facilities.

PHARMACISTS

Pharmacists provide consultation to, and dispense drugs ordered by, physicians and other practitioners. They understand drug biochemical properties, effective dosages, methods of administration, interactions, and side effects. Pharmacists also counsel patients about pharmaceuticals and their appropriate use.

There are eighty-two colleges of pharmacy in the United States with a total enrollment of twenty-nine thousand students; the number of graduates per year averages seventy-three hundred. Historically, there have been two types of pharmacy training programs: undergraduate (leading to award of a B.S. degree in pharmacy) and professional doctorate (leading to award of a Pharm.D. degree). Baccalaureate programs will be phased out by 2005. Pharm.D. programs are four years in length; students enter with at least two years of undergraduate study, but most have a college degree. After obtaining their Pharm.D. degree, some students pursue postgraduate (either M.S. or Ph.D.) programs preparing them for teaching and research roles; one- or two-year postgraduate residencies are available in areas of specialty practice.

There are 208,000 practicing pharmacists; 60 percent work in community pharmacies, retail chains, grocery stores, pharmaceutical wholesalers, or mass merchandisers; 20 percent are employed in hospitals. Their median income is $71,000.

OTHER HEALTH PROFESSIONALS

Here are five illustrations of other health professions. Three practice independently (chiropractors, optometrists, and podiatrists), while the other two typically work under the direction of a physician (physical therapists and physician assistants).

Chiropractors

Chiropractors diagnose and treat problems of the nervous, muscle, and skeletal systems, especially the spine. Chiropractic is based on the theory that obstruction in these systems, in addition to impairing functioning, lowers resistance to certain diseases. Practitioners provide drugless and nonsurgical treatments employing musculoskeletal adjustment and manipulation. Historically, allopathic medicine has challenged both the efficacy of chiropractic treatment and the theories on which it is based.

Chiropractors have a minimum of two years of undergraduate education (and increasingly, four), in addition to completing four years of chiropractic training. There are sixteen chiropractic colleges; no recent data are available on their enrollment. The first two years of education focus on basic sciences; the second two years entail course work in manipulative and adjustment techniques and training in clinical disciplines such as physical diagnosis, neurology, orthopedics, physiotherapy, and sports medicine. Graduation leads to award of the doctor of chiropractic (D.C.) degree. All practitioners must pass a state-administered examination before being granted a license to practice.

There are approximately fifty thousand professionally active chiropractors. Virtually all work in ambulatory settings, which are solo practices or partnerships. Chiropractors are rarely granted staff privileges in hospitals. Their average income is approximately $67,000.

Optometrists

Optometrists diagnose and treat vision problems and some ocular diseases. They perform vision tests and prescribe eyeglasses, contact lenses, and other treatments; they can also prescribe certain drugs. Optometrists should not be confused with either ophthalmologists or opticians. The former are physicians who provide a spectrum of medical and surgical eye care; the latter fit glasses according to the prescriptions of optometrists or ophthalmologists.

Optometrists typically have three or four years of undergraduate education in addition to four years of training in a school of optometry. Like other health professional schools, optometry education consists of two components:

study of the basic sciences and supervised clinical training. There are seventeen schools of optometry in the United States, with a total first year enrollment of approximately fourteen hundred students. Upon graduation, students must pass an exam before being granted a license to practice by the states.

There are approximately thirty thousand professionally active optometrists. All optometry care is provided on an outpatient basis. Practice sites and arrangements are diverse: independent solo and small group practice; and employment in retail vision care centers, medical groups, clinics, and hospitals. Their median annual income is $120,000.

Physical Therapists

Physical therapists focus on the musculoskeletal system and provide services that restore functioning, improve mobility, and prevent or limit disabilities. They treat patients through nondrug or surgical therapies such as exercise, stimulation, massage, ultrasound, adaptive devices (crutches and braces), and prostheses. Practitioners may be sought out directly by patients or referred by physicians.

As of 2002, all physical therapy training was required to be at the graduate level. There are 198 accredited programs; 165 offer a master's degree and 33 offer a doctorate. The curriculum includes training in the basic sciences, physical diagnosis and examination, and therapeutic procedures; classroom instruction is complemented by supervised clinical experience. All graduates are required to pass a licensing examination before they can practice. Doctoral programs prepare students for teaching and research positions, in addition to advanced practice in specialty areas such as pediatrics, geriatrics, orthopedics, sports medicine, neurology, and cardiopulmonary physical therapy.

There are approximately 144,000 professionally active physical therapists; 25 percent work part-time. Physical therapists are employed in hospitals, nursing homes, home health agencies, clinics, and physician offices (particularly those of orthopedic specialists); some are engaged in independent solo practice. Their median annual income is $55,000.

Physician Assistants

Physician assistants (P.A.s) provide a broad range of diagnostic and thera-peutic services. They take histories, conduct examinations, order and in-terpret tests, make diagnoses, and perform procedures (such as suturing, splinting, and casting); in all but three states they can prescribe certain med-ications. A P.A.'s practice must be linked to, and supervised by, a physician; however, it need not be immediate or direct. For example, in hospitals and clinics, P.A.s see patients without a physician being present; in rural areas they often function as primary care providers, consulting with supervising physicians by telephone and during periodic visits. Historically, the devel-opment of this profession was based on the training and practice of medics and pharmacist mates in the military.

There are 129 accredited P.A. training programs (with a total enrollment of about six thousand students), which award associate, baccalaureate, and master's degrees; training takes at least two years. Students receive classroom instruction in the basic sciences in addition to supervised clinical experience in hospitals and ambulatory care settings. All states require P.A. graduates to take a national certifying examination; after passing this exam they can use the PA-C credential (certified physician assistant). Postgraduate education programs (of variable length) are available in internal medicine, primary care, emergency medicine, surgery, pediatrics, and occupational medicine.

There are approximately forty thousand practicing P.A.s; 56 percent work in physician offices, medical groups, and clinics; 32 percent are employed by hospitals; half provide primary care and half engage in some form of specialty practice. One-third of all P.A.s provide primary care in commu-nities with fewer than fifty thousand residents. The median annual income of a full-time P.A. is $65,000.

Podiatrists

Podiatrists diagnose and treat diseases and injuries of the foot and lower leg in addition to providing preventive care. They take X rays, prescribe certain drugs, set fractures, apply casts, fit prosthetic devices, and perform surgery.

Entrants to the seven schools of podiatry (with a total enrollment of about two thousand students) typically possess an undergraduate degree. The training program, consisting of instruction in the basic sciences and supervised clinical training, lasts four years. Upon graduation, students are awarded a doctor of podiatric medicine (D.P.M.) degree. All states require successful completion of a written and oral examination before granting a license. Most graduates complete a one-year general residency prior to entering practice. Postgraduate training (lasting up to three years) is available in such areas as anesthesiology, pathology, radiology, emergency medicine, surgery, and sports medicine.

There are approximately twelve thousand practicing podiatrists, most of whom are solo practitioners; their median annual income is $107,000. Some hospitals grant podiatrists staff privileges.

CHAPTER 5

Predictions and Challenges

The previous four chapters have told it like it is, describing the U.S. health care industry at the dawn of the twenty-first century—the general characteristics, organizations, and services provided, as well as the finances and the workforce. We turn now to a more hazardous duty: making predictions and identifying challenges. Two anonymous quotes capture our predicament:

When looking into a crystal ball, be ready to eat cut glass.

The problems one identifies say far more about the beholder than about what is beheld.

The health care industry has been resilient, adaptive, and creative. Additionally, access and quality have been enviable. The old adage is true: if you are really sick, America is the place to be.

Still, be forewarned: the following pages focus on problems. But the industry's greatest opportunities lie in resolving them.

Governance. Far more will be expected of health care organization boards, for several reasons. First, thanks to changing industry economic dynamics and increased competition in most markets, health care organizations' survival, let alone their "thrival," is not ensured. The most important matters arrive at the boardroom door. Boards will be required to make crucial decisions that define the organizational future. Second, health care organizations are becoming larger and more complex enterprises. Boards must oversee enterprises with revenues in the hundreds of millions or billions of dollars. Third, in the post-Enron era, the "cross bar" of governance responsibility and accountability has risen dramatically. The expectations are being defined by new federal legislation such as the Sarbanes-Oxley Act (the most widely publicized provision requires CEOs and CFOs to attest to the accuracy of financial statements), rules being promulgated by the New York Stock Exchange, and principles employed by large pension and trust funds and endorsed by the National Association of Corporate Directors. Although presently they are applicable only to commercial corporations, most observers believe they will be extended to large nonprofit organizations. Increasingly, they will affect the governance expectations of bond-rating agencies and insurers, regulators and accrediting bodies, state attorneys general, major donors and grant organizations, and the public. As Alan Greenspan, chairman of the Federal Reserve, recently observed, "Board quality is the single best indicator of a corporation's character." Governance matters, and it will continue to do so more than ever before.

Aging of the population. Dramatic changes in demographics are a fundamental driver of major problems and opportunities that will be faced by our society in general and the health care industry in particular. Baby boomers begin turning sixty-five in 2010; in that year, the average life expectancy for males will be seventy-six and for females eighty-six. Biological and physical-based disease and infirmity, largely genetically programmed, increase exponentially with age. How this will be translated into demand for health care services is uncertain, given changes in lifestyles, biomedical and pharmacological technologies, the way health care is provided (for example, a shift from inpatient to outpatient and home care) and financing priorities (rationing care for certain population groups or conditions). Changing demographics is the health care industry's wild card. It will have a tremendous impact, but no one knows exactly what and how much.

Federal government initiatives. Major health care reform failed in the early 1990s, and future legislative efforts are unlikely to succeed; the one exception is Medicare (see below). National health insurance will not be implemented. No major programs to significantly expand federally mandated

The Health Care Industry: A Primer

or financed health care benefits will be undertaken. Expect continuous incremental change that limits federal government health care expenditures and makes health insurance plans (particularly HMOs) more accountable and patient-friendly.

Medicare. This is the industry's thousand-pound gorilla, the largest health plan and the biggest payer for hospital and physician services. Medicare's financial structure is untenable. In a status quo scenario, payroll tax contributions from employers and employees in addition to premiums paid by Part B beneficiaries will be less than expenditures; the gap will widen dramatically through 2010 and then go ballistic each year thereafter. There are only two alternatives. First, Medicare becomes bankrupt, which is highly unlikely given the importance of this program to a large segment of the population and the amount of political capital at stake. Second, Medicare is fundamentally and dramatically reconfigured. This entails some, or all, of the following: increasing age limits when benefits commence; increasing employer and employee payroll taxes and contributions; limiting coverage on the basis of need (implementing "means" tests to determine eligibility); restricting benefits; increasing co-insurance payments and deductibles; and further reducing payments to hospitals and physicians. Any or all of these changes will have significant implications for health care organizations and professionals.

Health insurance and health plans. Over the last several decades, the biggest change in how health care services are purchased has been the rapid growth of managed care, particularly HMO plans. HMO enrollment will continue to grow, but at a slower pace. However, HMOs will continue being dominant players. Other types of health plans will become more stringently "managed." Utilization and costs will be increasingly controlled. Additionally, there will be a growth in tiered health plans, where the array of benefits varies widely between higher- and lower-priced options.

Hospitals. Thanks to alterations in the industry's fundamental economic structure and dynamics, the majority of general, short-stay hospitals now have margins from operations that are in the red. This degree of financial distress will continue and is likely to get worse. With minimal internally generated reserves and inability to secure debt financing at reasonable rates, hospitals will find it increasingly difficult to modernize or replace facilities (whose half-life is eroding), mount or expand new programs and services, purchase and deploy innovative therapeutic and diagnostic technologies, and align wage rates for critical personnel with those in other industries.

Long-term care. Because of population aging, the increase of chronic disease, and the demise of extended families (who live close to one another and provide in-home care for their elderly), the need for all types of long-term care will increase dramatically throughout the first half of the twenty-first century. Whether this need is translated into demand for nursing home and home health care depends on financing. Most people do not have long-term care insurance. Private-pay nursing home care averages $50,000 per year, far beyond the means of all but the most well-to-do Americans. Medicare provides some long-term care benefits, but only after a hospital stay and then with strict limitations. Medicaid covers nursing home care, but one must exhaust one's resources before being eligible and payments to providers are low. Expect a fast-growing gap between what people need and want—and are able to afford—and the scope of services the system is able to provide.

Health systems. The promise of horizontally and vertically combined health systems has for the most part not materialized. Mergers and acquisitions have produced large, complex, and unwieldy organizations; cost reductions and economies of scale and scope have not been achieved; the purchase of physician practices and assuming first-dollar risk on providing services (that is, moving into the health insurance business) have produced huge losses; and true integration (of patient movement and clinical and management systems) has been problematic. There will be a slowdown in combinations to form health care systems. Additionally, an increasing number of systems will de-integrate, splitting into component parts. Those that survive (and there will be many) will have to demonstrate added clinical, strategic, and operational value.

Public health. HIV/AIDS, newly emerging viruses, antibiotic-resistant bacteria, increasing pollution of the environment, and threats of bioterrorism pose significant public health challenges. The public health system (actually a nonsystem) has been marginalized and is chronically underfunded, fragmented, overly bureaucratic, and focused on providing safety-net personal health care services. Absent a massive overhaul, the appropriateness and quality of public health services will continue to deteriorate.

Physicians. Doctors in the prime of their practice face a very different (and far less hospitable) environment than when they entered practice. Confronted with restrictions on clinical autonomy due to management of care, their base of patients is increasingly determined and controlled by health plans; the amount of red tape and paperwork with which they must contend to receive payment for their services is overwhelming. Additionally, there is a growing oversupply of physicians, although their distribution remains uneven among states, urban and rural locales, and individual markets. There are approximately 570,000 active physicians, with another 170,000 in the pipeline (medical students and residents); three new physicians appear for every one who retires. Having little control over industry-wide forces affecting them, many physicians feel disenfranchised.

Workforce. There will be increasing shortages of many types of health care professionals. For hospitals, the biggest problem is registered nurses (the largest, and most important, professional component of the hospital workforce). First, owing to the increasingly stringent management of care and the shift of many procedures to ambulatory care settings (such as same-day surgery), patients have shorter stays and require far more intense services (the so-called quicker-and-sicker phenomenon). Nursing bears most of the brunt. Second, the demand for R.N.s will outstrip supply at a growing rate. The average age of practicing R.N.s is forty-five, and increasing. More mature and experienced nurses are retiring, choosing to work part-time or moving into outpatient settings, where physical demands are less. Nursing school enrollment and graduation rates are flat because of a host of factors: a much expanded array of educational and employment opportunities for college-age women, changes in the structure of nursing education (toward a B.S.N. as the degree required for entry into practice), and no growth in real-dollar nursing salaries over the past several decades.

Biomedical technology. Major new medical technologies (devices, pharmaceuticals, and procedures) are being developed and introduced at a blistering pace. Many of these innovations are revolutionary and disruptive; that is, they will fundamentally alter, not just improve, clinical diagnostics and therapeutics. Technologies likely to have the greatest impact include:

- Genetic testing, employing maps of the human genome to identify predispositions for a host of diseases, conditions, and infirmities
- Gene therapy, using site-specific gene "implants" to change the course of, or eliminate, diseases
- Pharmaceuticals that will totally replace current forms of treatment; for example, "Drano-like" drugs that remove plaque from coronary arteries, to obviate implanting stints or doing bypass surgery
- Xeno-transplantation, using animal cells, tissues, and organs as a source for human transplants
- Minimally invasive procedures, accelerated development of devices and techniques that allow interventions to be performed without major surgery

These, and a host of other, developments will change how health care services are organized, provided, and reimbursed.

Information technology. Dramatic developments in computer, Internet-based, and communications technologies are sweeping across all sectors of the economy. In the health care industry, they will have a significant impact on how clinical and administrative information is collected, stored, analyzed, integrated, and used; the effectiveness, efficiency, and timeliness of internal operating systems; and how patients, purchasers, clinicians, and health care organizations interact with one another.

Plenty of challenges? You bet! How they are addressed, and the fate of the organization on whose board you serve, will depend on the quality of your board's governance. Seize the opportunity to make a difference!

Glossary of Health Care Terms

Like all fields, health care has its own specialized lingo, which can be confusing and overwhelming. Here are definitions of some key concepts, terms, and acronyms to help you begin navigating the terrain.

Adjusted patient days: An aggregate figure reflecting the volume of weighted inpatient and outpatient services provided by a hospital.

Administrative services organization (ASO): An organization (typically a component of an insurance company) that performs only administrative functions for an employer with a self-funded health plan. The employer assumes all risks associated with the provision of payments or services to beneficiaries.

Admission certification: A method of ensuring that only those patients needing care are admitted to a hospital. Approval can be granted either before admission (precertification) or shortly thereafter (concurrent certification). An authorization is typically assigned on the basis of the patient's diagnosis and prognosis.

Adverse selection: The tendency for individuals who have poor health status and a high utilization rate to purchase health insurance (or seek greater, and more comprehensive, coverage).

Affiliated (or contract) provider: A health care organization or professional that is part of a health plan's network; it contracts to provide services to the plan's members for a fee, set price, or capitated rate.

Affiliation: A form of cooperative agreement in which organizations coordinate their activities without merging.

Allowable cost: Provider costs that are deemed to be reimbursable under the payment formula of a health plan. For example, in calculating payments to hospitals Medicare specifies which cost types are allowable and which are not. The Centers for Medicare and Medicaid Services (CMS) publishes an extensive list of rules governing them. Disallowed costs are those deemed to be unnecessary for effective or efficient provision of care to beneficiaries.

All patient diagnosis related groups (APDRG): An enhancement of the original DRG methodology (see *diagnosis related group*) that applies to a population broader than Medicare beneficiaries. APDRGs, for example, include groupings for pediatric and maternity cases.

All payer system: A system of reimbursing providers in which prices for health services and payment methods are the same, regardless of who is paying. For example, federal or state government, a private insurer, a self-insured plan, and an individual all pay the same rate. The uniform fee negates the need of providers shifting costs from one payer to another.

Ambulatory (outpatient) care: Health services provided without the patient being admitted for an overnight stay in a hospital.

Ambulatory patient classifications (APC): A methodology for classifying ambulatory or outpatient services and procedures for purposes of payment by health plans. More than seven thousand services and procedures are grouped into about three hundred APCs.

Ambulatory surgery center: A facility where surgical procedures are performed on an outpatient basis. The facility may be freestanding or affiliated with a hospital.

Assignment of benefits: Arrangement where a beneficiary directs a health plan to make payments directly to a provider.

Assisted living facility: Homelike, residential facility that provides personal and basic nursing care for people who are aged, infirm, dependent, or experiencing mental or behavioral problems.

Average length of stay (ALOS): Number of days the average patient stays in a facility during a specific period of time. Calculated as the total number of patient days divided by the number of admissions.

Average daily census (ADC): The number of individuals in an inpatient facility (hospital, nursing home) on an average day; typically counted at midnight.

Balance billing: The practice of billing a patient for the fee remaining after insurer and copayments have been made. Under Medicare, the balance billed cannot exceed 15 percent of the total approved charge.

Beds, hospital: The average number of beds, cribs, and pediatric bassinets set-up and staffed on the last day of a given reporting period.

Behavioral health services: Diagnosis, treatment, and care of individuals with mental illness or chemical dependency. Services may be provided on an inpatient or outpatient basis and are performed by psychiatrists, psychologists, clinical social workers, or other licensed professionals.

Benchmark: A standard by which something is to be measured, compared, or judged. Benchmarking involves identifying best practices in peer organizations and then comparing one's performance to them.

Beneficiary: An individual eligible to receive benefits under a health plan.

Benefit package: A listing and description of benefits covered by a health plan.

Board, governing: The entity that bears ultimate fiduciary responsibility, accountability, and authority for an organization. The board is obligated to serve as an agent of stakeholders or shareholders and ensure the organization's resources and capacities are deployed in ways that benefit them.

Board-certified physician: A physician who has successfully completed a residency in addition to meeting the examination and practice requirements specified by one of twenty-four medical specialty boards.

Board-eligible physician: A physician who has successfully completed a residency program in one of twenty-four recognized medical specialties but who has not fulfilled practice and examination requirements.

Cafeteria employee benefit plan: Flexible plan where an employer provides a range of benefits options that can be chosen by employees on the basis of their needs or wants. Examples are life insurance, disability insurance, health insurance, dental insurance, vision care, legal services, child and dependent care, retirement plans, and vacation time.

Capitation (cap): The dollar amount paid periodically to a health provider for a contracted set of services delivered to a group of beneficiaries.

The provider is paid a fixed amount for each "covered life" or member irrespective of the number or nature of services provided. (see also *PMPM,* per member per month)

Carve-out benefits: Health care benefits that are provided and administered separately from a standard health plan. They might include mental health, substance abuse, vision, dental, and prescription drugs.

Case management: A method of planning and managing the services provided to an individual though a course of treatment in a cost-effective manner. It is intended to ensure provision of appropriate care in addition to reducing fragmentation and inappropriate utilization. Case managers are typically registered nurses.

Case mix (index): A measure of the complexity and resource requirements of patients treated by a particular provider.

Catastrophic health insurance: Insures the cost of treating severe or lengthy illness or disability. Generally such policies cover all, or a specified percentage of, medical expenses above an amount that is the responsibility of another (basic) health plan up to a maximum limit.

Centers for Medicare and Medicaid Services (CMS): Formerly the Health Care Financing Administration (HCFA). This is the federal government agency that administers the Medicare and Medicaid programs, conducts research to support them, and oversees more than a quarter of all health care expenditures in the United States.

Certificate of need (CON): In some states, approval that hospitals must seek (in specified instances) before building facilities, changing or enlarging services, or purchasing equipment.

Charge: Price set by a provider for a specific service. Full charges might not be paid by health plans thanks to discounts and deductions.

Chief executive officer (CEO): Individual responsible to a board for the strategic, fiscal, and operational management of an organization.

Chronic disease: A condition that does not improve and lasts the remainder of a person's life. It is manageable but cannot be totally cured and may be major (AIDS) or minor (gradual hearing loss).

Clinical (or critical) pathways (or protocols): A detailed description of the nature and sequencing of best treatment and intervention activities. The pathway or protocol outlines the type of information needed to make clinical decisions, the timing of treatments and procedures, and which actions need to be undertaken by whom. They are developed by clinicians for specific diseases or medical events.

Coordination of benefits: Provisions and procedures of health plans used to avoid duplicate payments when claims are covered by more than one company.

Complementary or alternative medicine: Health care services that complement traditional "Western" medical therapies, such as acupuncture, homeopathy, herbal medicine, massage, and meditation.

Consolidated Omnibus Budget Reconciliation Act (COBRA): A federal statute that requires employers to offer continued health plan benefits to certain employees and their dependents whose group coverage has been terminated. COBRA typically makes continued coverage available for up to thirty-six months. Enrollees may be required to pay 100 percent of the premium, plus an additional surcharge.

Community rating: A system of setting health plan premiums on the basis of the average cost of providing services to all individuals in a class of beneficiaries without adjusting for an individual's risk or utilization history.

Consumer price index (CPI): A measure of inflation in the prices of a standard "market basket" of goods and services.

Continuum of care: An array of health care services including preventive, ambulatory, acute inpatient, skilled nursing, rehabilitation, and home care.

Copayment: Provision of a health plan requiring an insured person to pay (out of pocket), at the time of service, a specified dollar amount or percentage of the fee. Examples are a charge of $10 every time a prescription is filled; or, under Medicare Part B (which covers physician services), paying 20 percent of allowed charges.

Cost: Estimated by accounting procedures, the dollar value of all resources consumed in producing a specific service.

Cost center: An accounting device whereby all related costs attributable to some department, unit, or program within a provider organization are segregated for accounting or reimbursement purposes.

Cost sharing: Occurs, for example, when both employees and employers contribute to health plan premium costs.

Cost shifting: A situation that occurs when providers reallocate costs from one payer group to another. When providers are not reimbursed, or fully reimbursed, for the costs of services (to the uninsured or to Medicare or Medicaid patients), charges to those who do pay are increased.

Covered lives: Group of individuals who are entitled to receive benefits or services under a health plan.

Customary, prevailing, and reasonable (CPR) charge: A method that was used to reimburse physicians under Medicare. Payment for a service was limited to the lowest of the physician's billed charge for the service, the physician's customary charge for the service, or the prevailing charge for that service in the community.

Deductible: The amount a beneficiary must pay out of pocket before a health plan's coverage is activated.

Defined benefits coverage: An approach to health insurance where employers promise to provide beneficiaries a specific package of services.

Defined contribution coverage: An approach to health insurance where employers make a specific dollar contribution toward the cost of insurance coverage for employees without defining or guaranteeing the nature or amount of services provided.

Diagnosis related groups (DRG): A patient classification system used by Medicare to pay hospitals for their services. The methodology groups patients into approximately five hundred homogeneous resource consumption categories that are based on their age, sex, principle and secondary diagnosis, procedure performed (if any), and discharge status.

Direct contracting: An arrangement whereby employers, unions, and other purchasers bypass health plans and contract directly with an organized provider network.

Disallowance: When a health plan declines to pay for all or part of a claim submitted by a provider.

Discounted fee-for-service: An arrangement where organizations and professionals agree to provide services to a health plan at a percentage discount from customary charges.

Disproportionate share hospital (DSH) adjustment: A payment adjustment for hospitals that serve a relatively large volume of low-income patients.

Drug formulary: A list of prescription drugs available in a hospital or approved by a health plan for their beneficiaries.

Durable medical equipment (DME): Nondisposable medical equipment that supplements the care process—such items as crutches, wheelchairs, beds, infusion pumps, and monitoring devices.

Economic credentialing: The use of economic criteria, unrelated to quality of care or professional competency, for determining a physician's qualifications for initial or continuing medical staff membership and privileges.

Exclusive provider arrangement (EPA): A health plan that provides benefits only if care is rendered by organizations and professionals with whom it contracts; there are typically exceptions for emergency and out-of-area services.

Evidence-based medicine: The conscientious, explicit, and judicious use of current best practices (based on empirical evidence regarding outcomes) when making decisions about the care of patients.

Experience rating: The process of setting health insurance premiums (in whole or part) on the basis of the historical claims or utilization experience of a particular group.

Federal Employees Health Benefits Program (FEHBP): The health plan for all federal employees, who can choose to participate in a service benefit plan administered by Blue Cross and Blue Shield or an indemnity plan offered by Aetna Life Insurance.

Fee-for-service: A traditional method of reimbursing providers for the services rendered to beneficiaries. The plan pays a fee (usually billed charges) for each specific service provided.

First dollar coverage: The health plan pays for all health care costs; beneficiaries have no deductible and make no copayments.

Fiscal intermediary: An entity, usually an insurance company, that makes payments to providers (and performs other administrative functions) on behalf of Medicare. Also called a third-party administrator (TPA).

Gatekeeper: A health care professional (typically primary care physician or nurse) responsible for determining the services a patient can use under a health plan.

Global budget: A national or state limit on the total amount of public and private expenditures for health care services.

Group health insurance: Health insurance purchased by, and provided to, a population of individuals—for example, all employees of a particular employer. The premium is calculated for the group as a whole (on the basis of age, sex, health status, and other risk factors).

Group model health plan: An arrangement where a health plan contracts with organized groups of physicians (partnerships or professional corporations) to provide services to beneficiaries.

Group practice: A group of physicians who engage in coordinated practice. This might include sharing facilities, equipment, supplies, and support personnel; consulting with one another in the care of patients; cross referring; and contracting with health plans.

Group purchasing organization (GPO): An organization that pools provider members (health systems and hospitals) and contracts for purchasing equipment, supplies, and services at discounted prices based on high volume. Typically, members must agree to make a specified amount of purchases through the GPO.

Health: Defined by the World Health Organization (WHO) as "complete physical, mental and social well-being . . . not merely the absence of disease or infirmity."

Health Insurance Purchasing Cooperatives (HIPCs): Organizations that secure health insurance coverage for a collection of groups (for instance, employers, local governments, associations) on a cooperative basis. The goal is to obtain greater leverage and lower prices when negotiating with health plans.

Health maintenance organization (HMO): A health plan that combines in one entity (through ownership or contract) insurance and provision functions. The plan contracts with purchasers to provide a comprehensive package of benefits at a capitated rate per member.

Health plan: Generic term employed to describe organizations that underwrite health insurance benefits and bear some (or a portion of) the risk for providing a package of services to beneficiaries. Health plans may be pure payers or they can finance/provide services (through owned or contracted networks).

HIPAA (Health Insurance Portability and Accountability Act): A federal law intended to improve the availability and continuity of health insurance coverage that places limits on exclusions for preexisting medical conditions, permits certain individuals to enroll for available group health care coverage when they lose other health coverage or have a new dependent, prohibits discrimination in group enrollment that is based on health status, guarantees the availability of health coverage to small employers, requires provision of nongroup coverage to certain individuals whose group coverage is terminated, and establishes requirements regarding the collection and use of patient information.

Health Plan Employer Data and Information Set (HEDIS): A set of performance measures that standardize how health plans report data to employers in five areas: quality, access and patient satisfaction, membership and utilization, finance, and management.

Health promotion: A discipline that seeks to help individuals alter their lifestyles to enhance their health status and well-being.

Home health: Health care and supportive services provided at an individual's residence, including nursing care, various types of therapy, and assistance with activities of daily living.

Horizontal integration: The combination of like health care organizations (for example, hospitals, or medical groups) into one corporation.

Hospice: An organization that provides medical and supportive care to individuals who are terminally ill and their families. A hospice can be a freestanding facility, unit of a hospital, or an independent program. Care can be provided on an inpatient or outpatient basis.

Hospital: American Hospital Association designation: Institution with at least six beds that provides general/special diagnostic and therapeutic services to patients staying longer than twenty-four hours.

Hospital, community: American Hospital Association designation: a nonfederal general or special hospital.

Hospital, general: An organization that provides general medical and surgical inpatient care to individuals requiring relatively short lengths of stay.

Hospital, special: An organization providing inpatient care to individuals with specific diseases or conditions; may be either short-term or long-term.

Hospitalist: A physician whose practice is devoted to treating patients in a hospital setting.

Incidence: The number of new cases of a particular problem, condition, or disease that arise in an area during a period of time in a specific population.

Indemnity insurance: A health plan that provides a stipulated cash payment for covered health care services without regard to the actual expenses incurred by the beneficiary. For example, a patient might be reimbursed $500 per day of hospital stay.

Independent practice association or organization (IPA or IPO): An organization that contracts with health plans on behalf of independent physicians who work in their own private offices and see other than "contracted for" patients. IPAs are typically paid capitated rates by health plans. Individual physicians guarantee they will provide a specified set of services for beneficiaries assigned to them and are paid under a variety of arrangements, including discounted fee-for-service, rate schedule, or capitation.

Indigent care: Health care services provided at no cost to individuals who cannot afford to pay; they do not have health insurance and are not covered by Medicare, Medicaid, or other public programs.

International medical graduate (IMG): A physician who graduated from a medical school outside of the United States. U.S. citizens who graduate from medical schools abroad are classified as IMGs. Formally referred to as foreign medical graduates (FMGs).

Joint Commission on the Accreditation of Healthcare Organizations (JCAHO): The organization that accredits hospitals and other health care providers. The commission conveys accreditation on the basis of recommendations of a clinical or administrative site visit team that reviews policies, patient records, professional credentialing procedures, governance, and quality improvement programs.

Joint venture: A legal entity where two or more parties work together, sharing profits and losses; usually limited to a single project.

Licensed practical or vocational nurse (LPN/LVN): An individual who performs a variety of nonprofessional nursing functions, such as providing personal care; taking temperatures, blood pressure, pulse and respiration; recording results on charts; and observing a patient's condition. One year of formal education is required, typically gained in a community college or vocational institute.

Malpractice insurance: Insurance against the risk of incurring financial loss due to professional misconduct or lack of ordinary skill.

Management services organization (MSO): An organization that provides management services, systems, and support to one or more medical practices.

Medical group, foundation model: Organizational arrangement where a health system or hospital forms a tax-exempt entity that acquires the assets of a medical group and contracts with it for provision of professional services. The foundation typically employs all nonphysician personnel and is responsible for management, finances, contracting, facilities, equipment, and support services. The contracting medical group remains independent (the group is generally organized as a professional corporation).

Medicaid (Title XIX of the Social Security Act): A welfare program (established in 1966 through an amendment of the Social Security Act) that provides medical benefits to low-income persons in need of health care. Subject to broad federal guidelines, individual states determine benefits covered, program eligibility, rates of payment for providers, and methods of administering the program.

Medicare (Title XVIII of the Social Security Act): A federal program that provides health insurance to the elderly and certain disabled individuals, regardless of their financial status. Enacted in 1966 through an amendment to the Social Security Act, it consists of two separate but coordinated programs: hospital insurance (Part A) and supplementary medical insurance (Part B). Part A benefits are financed by payroll deductions. Part B benefits are financed by a combination of enrollee premiums and general tax funds.

Medigap insurance: A health plan that supplements Medicare coverage. Benefits may include payment of deductibles, coinsurance, and balance billings, as well as services not covered.

Morbidity: A measure of the incidence or prevalence of disease or disability in a particular population over a specified period of time.

Market share: A measure of the extent to which a provider has penetrated a particular market. It is calculated as the volume of a particular provider or service divided by the total volume of all providers (in a given market).

Mortality: A measure of the number of deaths in a particular population over a specified period of time.

National Practitioner Data Bank: A data repository maintained by the federal government that collects information on physicians against whom malpractice claims have been paid or disciplinary actions have been taken.

Open enrollment period: A designated period of time during which employees are permitted to change enrollment from one health plan to another offered by their employer.

Out-of-pocket expenditures: Payments made by consumers directly to providers for copayments, deductibles, balance billings, and noncovered services.

Outpatient visit: An occasion of service provided by a hospital to patients not requiring an overnight stay.

Peer review organization (PRO): Private organizations contracting with CMS (Centers for Medicare and Medicaid Services) to review the medical necessity and quality of services provided to Medicare beneficiaries.

Per diem rate: A form of payment where a hospital or nursing home is paid a set daily fee regardless of the cost of providing care.

Periodic interim payment: A regular payment made by a health plan to a provider that approximates anticipated revenue and is adjusted periodically to conform to actual revenues to assure predictable cash flow.

Per member per month (PMPM): Capitated payments made by a health plan to a provider for a specified set of services rendered to a beneficiary for the month of enrollment.

Pharmacy benefit manager (PBM): An organization that contracts with a health plan, HMO, or self-insured employer to manage and provide drug benefits.

Physician: Individual with an M.D. (doctor of medicine) or D.O. (doctor of osteopathy) degree licensed by states to practice the profession of medicine.

Physician-hospital organization (PHO): An organization owned by, and representing, a hospital and physicians (typically members of the hospital's medical staff). It serves as a hospital or physician agent for contracting with health plans.

Point-of-service plan (POS): A health plan where beneficiaries can choose among delivery systems (HMO, PPO, fee-for-service) when accessing services, rather than making the selection at the time of enrollment. The out-of-pocket expenses associated with receiving care from in-network providers is less than when care is rendered by noncontracting ones. Such a plan allows greater choice but imposes financial penalties for out-of-network usage.

Portability: The ability to move health insurance benefits from one employer to another without any disruptions or limitations in coverage.

Preferred provider organization (PPO): A combination of hospitals and physicians contracting with a health plan to provide a specific package of health care services to its beneficiaries. The PPO may be paid under a variety of financial arrangements, including capitation, fee schedule, or discounted fee-for-service.

Premium: The amount paid to a health plan (by an individual or purchaser) for providing coverage.

Prevalence: The number of existing cases of a particular disease or condition in a specific population during a given period of time.

Professional corporation (PC): A legal entity whose shareholders must be licensed members of the same profession; it entails limited liability for its professional stockholder(s) and allows corporate ownership of tangible and intangible assets.

Public health: A discipline that seeks to promote health and prevent disease in populations. The focus is on such things as immunization, sanitation, detection and control of communicable diseases, environmental hazards, and health education.

Relative value unit (RVU): A weight assigned to any of various medical services and procedures that reflect their complexity and resource intensity. The RVU is multiplied by a dollar conversion factor to determine payment to providers.

Revenue, deductions: The difference between revenue at full rates (charges) and the payment actually received.

Revenue, net patient: The amount of funds received from patients, third-party payers, and others for all services rendered.

Revenue, net total: Net patient revenue plus all other income, including contributions, endowment, grants, and other payments not made on behalf of individual patients.

Safe harbor: A set of federal regulations providing protection (criminal and civil) for certain health care business practices entered into by hospitals and physicians when specified requirements are met.

Sentinel event: A term used by the JCAHO to define an adverse patient occurrence in an accredited facility.

Skilled nursing facility: An organization that provides residential, non-acute medical and nursing care, therapy, and social services under the direction of a registered nurse on a twenty-four-hour basis.

Sole community provider: A health care facility located in an isolated area that serves as the only source of emergency, outpatient, and in-patient care in the region. These facilities receive a special designation from CMS and a different payment formula that provides greater reimbursement.

Staff model HMO: A type of health maintenance organization where all or most medical services to beneficiaries are provided by physician employees.

Swing beds: Acute care hospital beds that can also be used for long-term care patients.

Teaching hospital: A hospital, typically affiliated with a medical school, that offers accredited medical residency training programs.

Telemedicine: The use of computer and Internet technology for delivering health care services.

TRICARE: A federally sponsored health plan for military veterans and their dependents (formerly called CHAMPUS).

Uncompensated care: Services provided by hospitals and physicians for which no payment is received from either the patient or the health plan.

Underinsured: Individuals who may have public or private health insurance but whose coverage is limited or minimal.

Uniform hospital discharge data set: A set of data elements that describe a hospital inpatient stay: age, sex, race, residence, length of stay, diagnosis, procedures performed, disposition, and source of payment.

Usual, customary, and reasonable (UCR): Typical fees charged for the provision of specific health care services in a particular area on the basis of the provider's usual charge or amount customarily charged by other providers in an area.

Utilization review (UR): Evaluation of the necessity, appropriateness, effectiveness, and efficiency of services, procedures, and facilities employed to care for patients.

Vertical integration: The combination of organizations where the output of one is the input of another—for example, consolidating a hospital, medical group, and nursing home.

Workers' compensation: A state-mandated program providing health insurance coverage for work-related injuries and disabilities.

Medical Specialties

Allergy and immunology: Evaluation, diagnosis, and treatment of immune system disorders. Training required: two years in addition to prior certification in internal medicine or pediatrics. Subspecialty certification is available in clinical and laboratory immunology.

Anesthesiology: Provision of pain relief and maintenance or restoration of a stable condition during an operation or diagnostic procedure. Training required: four years postmedical school. Subspecialty certification is available in critical care medicine and pain management.

Colon and rectal surgery: Diagnosis and treatment of diseases of the intestinal tract, colon, rectum, anal canal, and perianal area. Training required: six years, including completion of a residency in general surgery.

Dermatology: Diagnosis and treatment of patients with benign and malignant conditions of the skin, mouth, external genitalia, hair, and nails, as well as a number of sexually transmitted diseases. Training required: four years postmedical school. Subspecialty certification is available in clinical or laboratory dermatological immunology and dermathopathology.

Emergency medicine: Evaluation, care, stabilization, and disposition of patients with acute illness and injury, typically in a hospital emergency room. Training required: three years postmedical school. Subspecialty certification is available in medical pathology, pediatric emergency medicine, and sports medicine.

Family practice: Provision of total health care to individuals and families, including diagnosis and treatment of a variety of ailments in patients of all ages. Training required: three years postmedical school. Subspecialty certification is available in geriatric medicine and sports medicine.

Internal medicine: Provision of nonsurgical, comprehensive ambulatory and hospital care to adolescents, adults, and the elderly. Training required: three years postmedical school. Subspecialty certification is available in adolescent medicine; cardiovascular disease; clinical cardiac electro-physiology; clinical and laboratory medicine; critical care medicine; endocrinology, diabetes, metabolism; gastroenterology; geriatric medicine; hematology; infectious diseases; interventional cardiology; medical oncology; nephrology; pulmonary disease; rheumatology; and sports medicine.

Medical genetics: Diagnosis and treatment of patients with genetically linked diseases. Training required: two to four years postmedical school. Subspecialty certification is available in medical genetics pathology.

Neurological surgery: Diagnosis, evaluation, treatment, and rehabilitation of patients with disorders of the central, peripheral, and autonomic nervous systems. Training required: seven years postmedical school (including completion of a residency in general surgery).

Neurology: Diagnosis and nonsurgical treatment of diseases and impaired functioning of the brain, spinal cord, peripheral nerves, muscles, and autonomic nervous system, including associated blood vessels. Training required: four years postmedical school. Subspecialty certification is available in clinical neurophysiology, neurodevelopmental disabilities, and pain management.

Nuclear medicine: Use of radioactive materials in diagnosing and treating disease. Training required: three years postmedical school.

Obstetrics and gynecology: Medical and surgical care focused on the female reproductive system and associated disorders. Members of this specialty typically serve as primary physicians for women. Training required: four years postmedical school. Subspecialty certification is available in critical care medicine, gynecologic oncology, maternal-fetal medicine, and reproductive endocrinology.

Ophthalmology: Diagnosis and treatment (through both medical and surgical means) of ocular and visual disorders, including diseases affecting the eye and its component structures, the eyelids, the orbit, and the visual pathway. Training required: four years postmedical school.

Orthopedic surgery: Preservation and restoration of the form and function of the extremities, spine, and associated structures by medical, surgical, and physical means. Training required: five years postmedical school (including a residency in general surgery). Subspecialty certification is available in hand surgery.

Otolaryngology: Medical and surgical care of patients with diseases and disorders that affect the ears, nose, throat, sinuses, respiratory and upper alimentary systems, face, jaws, and the head and neck. Training required: five years postmedical school. Subspecialty certification is available in otology or neurotology, pediatric otolaryngology, and plastic surgery within the head and neck.

Pathology: Deals with the causes and nature of disease and contributes to diagnosis and treatment through knowledge gained by laboratory application of the biologic, chemical, and physical sciences. Training required: five to seven years postmedical school. Subspecialty certification is available in blood bank and transfusion medicine, chemical pathology, cytopathology, dermatopathology, forensic pathology, hematology, medical microbiology, molecular genetic pathology, neuropathology, and pediatric pathology.

Pediatrics: Deals with the physical, emotional, and social health of children from birth through young adulthood, ranging from preventive health care to diagnosis and treatment of acute and chronic diseases. Training required: three years postmedical school. Subspecialty certification is available in adolescent medicine, clinical or laboratory immunology, developmental-behavioral pediatrics, medical toxicology, neonatal-perinatal medicine, neurodevelopmental disabilities, pediatric cardiology, pediatric critical care medicine, pediatric emergency medicine, pediatric endocrinology, pediatric gastroenterology, pediatric hematology-oncology, pediatric infectious diseases, pediatric nephrology, pediatric pulmonology, pediatric rheumatology, and sports medicine.

Physical medicine and rehabilitation: Diagnosis, evaluation, and treatment of patients with physical disabilities that arise from conditions affecting the musculoskeletal system or from neurological trauma or disease. Training required: four years postmedical school. Subspecialty certification is available in pain management, pediatric rehabilitation medicine, and spinal cord injury medicine.

Plastic surgery: Repair and reconstruction of physical defects involving the skin, musculoskeletal system, cranio-maxillofacial structures, hands, extremities, breasts, trunk, and external genitalia. Training required: five to seven years postmedical school. Subspecialty certification is available in plastic surgery within the head and neck and hand surgery.

Preventive medicine: Focuses on the health of individuals and defined populations to protect, promote, and maintain health and well-being, and to prevent disease, disability, and premature death. Many of these practitioners also hold an M.P.H. degree in public health. Training required: three years postmedical school. Subspecialty certification is available in medical toxicology and undersea or hyperbaric medicine.

Psychiatry: Prevention, diagnosis, and treatment of mental, behavioral, emotional, and addictive disorders. Training required: four years postmedical school. Subspecialty certification is available in addiction psychiatry, child and adolescent psychiatry, clinical neurophysiology, forensic psychiatry, geriatric psychiatry, and pain management.

Radiology: Use of emission technologies (particle, magnetic, and sound) to diagnose and treat disease. Training required: four years postmedical school. Subspecialty certification is available in neuroradiology, nuclear radiology, pediatric radiology, and vascular-interventional radiology.

Surgery (general): Management of a spectrum of diseases in all areas of the body requiring surgical intervention. Training required: five years postmedical school. Subspecialty certification is available in pediatric surgery, hand surgery, surgical critical care, and vascular surgery.

Thoracic surgery: Provision of operative, perioperative care, and critical care of patients with pathologic conditions in the chest. Training required: five years postmedical school.

Urology: Medical and surgical management of disorders involving the genitourinary system and adrenal gland. Training required: five years postmedical school.

Recommendations for Learning More

This book focuses on the health care industry, organizations and the services they provide, finances, and personnel—but gives little attention to governance. To learn more about health care organization boards and their work, we recommend:

Board Work, by Dennis Pointer and James Orlikoff (San Francisco: Jossey-Bass, 1999); winner of the James A. Hamilton Book of the Year Award from the American College of Healthcare Executives.
Getting to Great: Principles of Health Care Organization Governance, by Dennis Pointer and James Orlikoff (San Francisco: Jossey-Bass, 2002).

These two books can be ordered by calling (888) 378–2537 or logging on to www.josseybass.com.

To broaden and deepen your understanding of the health care industry, we recommend:

Introduction to Health Services, 6th ed., by Stephen Williams and Paul Torrens (Albany, N.Y.: Delmar, 2002).

This is the most widely used textbook in health administration programs for introducing graduate students to the industry's configuration and functioning. It can be ordered by calling (800) 730–2214 or logging on to www.delmar.com.

One of the industry's biggest challenges is ensuring the quality of care. Every health care organization board member should read:

To Err Is Human: Building a Safer Health System (Washington, D.C.: National Academy Press, Institute of Medicine, 2000).
Crossing the Quality Chasm: A New Health System for the 21st Century (Washington, D.C.: National Academy Press, Institute of Medicine, 2001).

You can learn more about these two significant studies, and read summaries of them, by logging on to the Institute of Medicine's Website at www.nas.edu/iom.

If you are a "data junkie" and want to see the detail for yourself, the best sources are:

Chartbook on Trends in the Health of Americans (Hyattsville, Md.: National Center for Health Statistics, 2002).
Health, United States—2002 (Hyattsville, Md.: Center for Health Statistics, 2002).

Both can be downloaded, free of charge, as PDF files at www.cdc.gov/nchs/hus.

The Internet is a gateway to a vast repository of information about everything. Web addresses (URLs), particularly references to specific pages, constantly change, so any listing becomes quickly dated. However, here are some particularly useful Websites as of the time of this writing:

Governance

American Governance and Leadership Group: www.americangovernance.com

National Center for Nonprofit Boards: www.boardsource.org

National Association of Corporate Directors: www.nacdonline.org

Health Care Organizations and Services

American Hospital Association: www.aha.org

Joint Commission on Accreditation of Healthcare Organizations: www.jcaho.org

American Health Care Association (nursing home and long-term care): www.ahca.org

National Association for Home Care: www.nahc.org

National Mental Health Association: www.nmha.org

American Association of Integrated Healthcare Delivery Systems: www.aaihds.org

American Public Health Association: www.apha.org

Health Care Financing

Centers for Medicare and Medicaid Services: www.hcfa.gov

Health Resources and Services Administration: www.hrsa.dhhs.gov

Health Insurance Association of America: www.hiaa.org

Blue Cross and Blue Shield Association: www.bluecares.com

Alliance of Community Health Plans: www.achp.org

Health Care Workforce

Bureau of Labor Statistics: www.bls.gov

Bureau of Health Professions: www.hrsa.gov/bhpr

American College of Healthcare Executives: www.ache.org

American Medical Association: www.ama-assn.org

American Osteopathic Association: www.aoa-net.org

American Nurses Association: www.nursingworld.org

American Dental Association: www.ada.org

American Pharmaceutical Association: www.aphanet.org

Other

Agency for Health Policy and Research: www.ahcpr.gov

Centers for Disease Control and Prevention (CDC): www.cdc.gov

Department of Health and Human Services: www.os.dhhs.gov

Fed Stats (home page for accessing government-compiled data): www.fedstats.gov

REFERENCES

We chose not to pepper the text with citations and footnotes. But we have drawn on a number of sources referred to here.

Unless otherwise noted, all data are from government sources in the public domain. Here are the sources most often used in this book:

Chartbook on Trends in the Health of Americans. Hyattsville, Md.: National Center for Health Statistics, 2002.
Health, United States—2002. Hyattsville, Md.: Center for Health Statistics, 2002.
Statistical Abstract of the United States, 2001. Washington, D.C.: U.S. Census Bureau, 2001.

Data in various sections and exhibits may, in some instances, not be perfectly consistent because they are taken from different sources. Additionally, data and percentages may not total perfectly, because of rounding.

Chapter 1

The four-stage evolutionary model is based on work of Perrow, C. "Goals and Power Structures: A Historical Analysis." In E. Freidson (ed.), *The Hospital in Modern Society.* London: Free Press of Glencoe, 1963.

Figures on the number of hospitals are taken from Quintana, J. B. "Hospital Governance and the Corporate Revolution." *Health Care Management Review,* 1985, *10*(3).

Data on health care systems and hospital boards are from studies conducted by Dennis D. Pointer for the Governance Institute in the late 1990s.

The sample consisted of 124 nonprofit, nongovernmental health systems drawn from subscribers of the Governance Institute, in addition to those listed in the *American Hospital Association Guide*, and 105 general hospitals that were Governance Institute subscribers.

Chapter 2

Source of data on ambulatory care utilization: various summaries in *National Ambulatory Care Survey*. Hyattsville, Md.: National Center for Health Statistics, 2001.

Data on physician groups were adapted from *Medical Groups in the U.S.: A Survey of Practice Characteristics*. Chicago: American Medical Association, 1999.

Source of data on community hospitals (Table 2.4): *Hospital Statistics*. Chicago: American Hospital Association, 2001.

General reference is made to Evashwick, C. "The Continuum of Long-Term Care." In S. Williams and P. Torrens (eds.), *Introduction to Health Services* (6th ed.). Albany, N.Y.: Delmar, 2002.

Source of data on nursing homes: *The Nursing Home Source Book*. Washington, D.C.: American Health Care Association, 2001.

Source of data on home health: *A Profile of Medicare Home Health, Chart Book*. Washington, D.C.: Health Care Financing Administration, 1999); and "Home Health On-Line," www.nahc.org (National Association for Home Care).

Torrens, P., and Breslow, L. "The Evolution of Public Health: A Joint Public-Private Responsibility," In Williams and Torrens (2002).

Scutchfield, F. D., and Keck, C. W. (eds.). *Principles of Public Health Practice*. Albany, N.Y.: Delmar, 2002.

Chapter 3

General reference: *Source Book of Health Insurance Data*. Washington, D.C.: Health Insurance Institute of America, 2000.

Data on health insurance coverage is from *Health Insurance Coverage*. Washington, D.C.: U.S. Census Bureau, 2000; and *Health Insurance Coverage and the Uninsured.* Washington, D.C.: Health Insurance Institute of America, 1999.

Data adapted from *Source Book of Health Insurance Data.* Washington, D.C.: Health Insurance Institute of America, 2000.

Chapter 4

Career Guide to Industries. Washington, D.C.: Bureau of Labor Statistics, 2001; *Occupational Outlook Handbook, 2001.* Washington, D.C.: Bureau of Labor Statistics, 2001; *Statistical Abstract of the United States.* Washington, D.C.: Bureau of the Census, 2001.

Levine, L. *A Shortage of Registered Nurses: Is It on the Horizon or Already Here?* Washington, D.C.: Congressional Research Service, Library of Congress, 2001.

Appendix A

Drawn from a variety of sources over the last decade, and adapted by Dennis Pointer for use in preparing course support materials.

Appendix B

Adapted from *Which Medical Specialty for You?* Evanston, Ill.: American Board of Medical Specialties, Research and Educational Foundation, 2000.

INDEX

Horizontal systems, 35–37, 88, 102. *See also* Health care systems
Hospices, 102
Hospitalist, 103
Hospitals, 24–27; boards of, 5, 12, 14–15, 27; closed- *versus* open-staff, 64; community, 26–27, 28, 102; defined, 102; dentists in, 80; expenditures for, 24–25; financial problems of, 87–88; future trends and, 87–88; general, 3–4, 25, 26–26, 28, 87, 103; in health maintenance organizations (HMOs), 63–65; historical evolution of, 2, 5–8, 24; long-term, 25; Medicare funding to, 59; mental health care in, 34, 35; nonprofit, 26; nurses in, 78, 89; operating and financial statistics for, 28; ownership of, 26–27; personnel in, 25, 27, 28; proprietary, 26; psychiatric, 4, 35; short-term, 3–4, 25, 26–27, 28, 88; specialty, 25–26, 103; statistical overviews of, 3–4, 25, 28; structural components of, 27, 29; types of, 25–26, 102–103; utilization rates of, 28

I

Idaho, physicians in, 73
Incidence, defined, 103
Income level: chiropractors', 81; dentists', 79; nurses', 78, 79; optometrists', 82; patients, utilization and, 12; pharmacists', 80; physical therapists', 82; physician assistants', 83; physicians', 72; podiatrists', 84. *See also* Economic status; Poverty
Indemnity plans, 52, 54, 103
Independent practice association (IPA) model HMO, 63–64, 67
Independent practice associations (IPAs), 103
Indian Health Service, 39
Indigent care, defined, 103
Individual providers, 1
Infant mortality rate, 9
Information technology, 90

Institute of Medicine, 118
Institutional providers, 1
Intensity, service, 47
Internal medicine, 76, 112
International medical graduate (IMG), 104
Intimacy, 18
Introduction to Health Services (Williams and Torrens), 117
Iowa, physicians in, 73

J

Japan, health care expenditures of, 42
Joint Commission on Accreditation of Healthcare Organizations (MCAHO), 2, 104, 109
Joint ventures, 37, 104

K

Kaiser Foundation Health Plan, 65
Kaiser Permanente Medical Group, 65
Knowles, J., 6

L

Leases, 37
Licensed practical nurses (L.P.N.s), 78–79, 104
Licensed vocational nurses (L.P.N.s), 78–79, 104
Licensing and certification: chiropractic, 81; dentist, 79; nurse, 76, 78; optometrist, 82; organizations of, 2; physician, 75; physician assistant, 83; podiatric, 84; specialty, 111–115
Life expectancy rates, 9
Limitations, 59
Local governments, 38; funding by, 47; public health in, 39–40
Long-term care, 27, 29–32; future trends and, 88; home health, 31–32; nursing home, 30–31
Louisiana, health insurance coverage in, 52

M

Malpractice insurance, 104
Managed care: contractual relationships in, 55–56; future growth of, 87; health

maintenance organization (HMO), 63–67; physician autonomy and, 89; structure of, 55–56. *See also* Health maintenance organizations (HMOs)

Management: governance and, 16, 27; hospital, 27

Management services organizations (MSOs), 104

Managers, 70

Market share, 105

Marx, K., 17–18

Maryland, physicians in, 72

Massachusetts, 39; physicians in, 72

Massachusetts General Hospital, 6

Medicaid, 61–63, 105; ambulatory care visits and, 22; coverage by, 61–62; enactment of, 7, 61, 105; home health agencies and, 32; industry financing and, 45; local public health and, 39; nursing homes and, 30, 31, 88; as public welfare insurance, 50, 61–63; uninsured population and, 51

Medical genetics, 112

Medical group, foundation model, 104–105

Medical inflation, 46

Medical school, 73–74, 104. *See also* Education, medical

Medical technology, 90

Medicare, 59–61, 105; allowable cost in, 92; ambulatory care visits and, 22; balance billing under, 93; coverage by, 59–60; enactment of, 7, 59, 105; financing of, 60, 61, 87; fiscal intermediaries and, 100; future of, 86–87; home health agencies and, 31–32; industry financing and, 45; local public health and, 39; nursing homes and, 30, 31, 88; Part A, 60–61, 105; Part B, 61, 87, 97, 105; physician reimbursement under, 60–61, 97–98; as social health insurance, 50, 59–61

Medigap insurance, 105

Mental and behavioral health, 33–35, 93–94; funding sources for, 33, 34; statistical overviews of, 4, 34–35

Mergers, 88

Minimally invasive procedures, 90

Minnesota, health insurance coverage in, 52

Mississippi, physicians in, 73

Mixed-model HMOs, 65, 67

Morbidity, defined, 105

Mortality, 106. *See also* Death

Multispecialty group practices, 23

N

National Ambulatory Care Survey, 21–23

National Association of Corporate Directors, 86

National Board Dental Examination, 79

National Center for Health Statistics, 21–23, 38, 118

National health insurance, 86

National Institutes of Health, 2, 38

National Practitioner Data Bank, 106

Need: demand and utilization and, 8, 10–12; services and, 18

Neurological surgery, 112

Neurology, 76, 112–113

New Hampshire, health insurance coverage in, 52

New Mexico, health insurance coverage in, 52

New York, physicians in, 72

New York Hospital, 2

New York Stock Exchange, 86

Nonprofit organizations: HMO, 65; home health, 32; hospital, 26

Nuclear medicine, 113

Nurses, 20, 75–79; advanced practice, 78; ancillary (L.P.N. and L.V.N.), 78–79, 104; distribution of, by practice setting, 77–78; education of, 75–77, 78, 89; future trends and, 89; income of, 78, 79; number of, 71, 77, 79, 89; statistical overview of, 4, 75–78. *See also* Registered nurses

Nursing homes: dentists in, 80; future trends and, 88; long-term care and, 30–31, 88; nurses in, 78, 79; statistical overviews of, 4, 30–31

Medicare funding to, 59; number of, 70–72; O.D., 72, 74; practice arrangements of, 23–24; statistical overview of, 4, 70–73; by type of practice, 72, 73; types of, 72, 111–115

Plastic surgery, 76, 114

Podiatrists, 20, 83–84; education of, 84; income of, 84; number of, 71, 84; overview of, 4, 83–84

Point-of-service plan (POS), 107

Pointer, D., 117

Policy development, in public health, 38

Population aging, 86, 88

Population covered by health insurance. See Health insurance coverage and status

Population growth, 47

Portability, 107

Poverty: health and disease status and, 10; Medicaid coverage and, 62; uninsured population and, 51, 53. See also Economic status; Income level

Predictions, for health care industry, 85–90

Preferred provider organization (PPO), 107

Premium, defined, 107

Prevalence, defined, 108

Preventive medicine specialty, 115

Preventive services, 22

Private initiatives, for public health care, 40

Professional associations, 2; Websites of, 118–120

Professional corporation (PC), 108

Professionalization, 19

Professionals, 69, 70–84; ambulatory care, 20–21; distribution of, 71; future trends and, 89; hospital, 27. See also Chiropractors; Dentists; Nurses; Optometrists; Personnel; Pharmacists; Physical therapists; Physician assistants; Physicians; Podiatrists; Providers; Workforce

Proprietary organizations: home health, 32; hospital, 26

Provider availability, utilization and, 12

Provider reimbursement, under Medicare, 60–61, 97–98

Providers: affiliated, 92; health insurance plan types and, 52, 54–56; in health maintenance organizations (HMOs), 63–65. See also Personnel; Professionals; Workforce

Psychiatry, 76, 115

Psychologists, 21

Public health, defined, 108

Public health care organizations and services, 17, 37–40; challenges to, 88–89; federal, 38–39; functions of, 37–38; future trends and, 88–89; local, 39–40; nurses in, 78; private initiatives for, 40; sector of, 1; state, 39. See also Health care organizations

Public welfare insurance, 50, 61–63. See also Medicaid

Purchasers, 19; health insurance plan types and, 52, 54–56; trends in characteristics of, 44, 45

Q

Quality assurance: governance and, 16; public health and, 38; resources on, 118

R

Race and ethnicity: access to ambulatory care and, 21; board composition and, 14; health and disease status by, 9; health insurance coverage and, 53; of M.D. medical students, 74; Medicaid coverage by, 62; of nursing home residents, 31; of registered nurses, 77; utilization and, 12, 13

Radiology, 76, 115

"Reasonable and customary" charges, 61

Referral patterns, utilization and, 12

Refuge state, 2, 5

Registered nurses (R.N.s): education of, 75–77, 89; future trends and, 89; number of, 71, 77, 89; overview of, 4, 75–78

and, 89; public health and, 88–89;
workforce challenges and, 89
TRICARE, 109

U

Uncompensated care, 109
Undergraduate medical education, 73–74
Uniform hospital discharge data set, 110
Uninsured population, 4, 50–52, 53, 110;
factors in growth of, 51–52, 53
United Kingdom, health care expenditures of, 42
U.S. Census Bureau, 17, 51
Urban areas, utilization in, 13
Urology, 76, 115
Usual, customary, and reasonable (UCR),
110
Utilization: factors in, 8, 10–12, 13, 18–19;
hospital, 28; key determinants of, 11;
percentage of population with no, 13
Utilization review (UR), 110

V

Vertical systems, 35–37, 88, 110. *See also*
Health care systems

Veterans Administration: as funding source,
47; mental health facilities of, 35
Voluntary health insurance (VHI), 50,
57–59

W

Websites, health-care-related, 118–120
Williams, S., 117
Workers' compensation, 22, 110
Workforce, health care industry: employment of, by organization type, 71;
future trends and, 89; in hospitals, 25;
jobs in, 69–70; professional nature of,
19; professionals in, 69, 70–84; professions *versus* occupations in, 69; statistical overview of, 4, 69–70; websites
about, 119. *See also* Personnel; Professionals; Providers
Workload, physician, 72
World Health Organization (WHO), 8,
101
Wyoming, physicians in, 73

X

Xeno-transplantation, 90